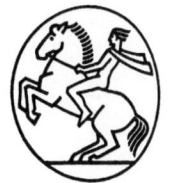

Metipranolol

Pharmacology of Beta-blocking
Agents and Use of
Metipranolol in Ophthalmology

Contributions to the First
Metipranolol Symposium, Berlin 1983

Edited by H.-J. Merté

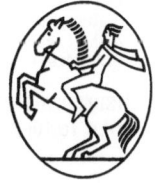

Springer-Verlag Wien GmbH

Prof. Dr. Hanns-Jürgen Merté

Director of the Eye Infirmary and Outpatient Eye Clinic rechts der Isar —
Technical University, Munich, Federal Republic of Germany

Translation of
"Metipranolol. Pharmakologie der Betablocker und ophthalmologische
Anwendung von Metipranolol"
Wien - New York: Springer. 1983
© 1983 by Springer-Verlag/Wien

© 1984 by Springer-Verlag Wien
Originally published by Springer- Verlag Wien New York in 1984

With 73 Figures (1 in colour)

Library of Congress Cataloging in Publication Data. Metipranolol Symposium (1st : 1983 : Berlin,
Germany). Metipranolol: pharmacology of beta-blocking agents and use of metipranolol in ophthalmology. Translation of: Metipranolol. 1. Glaucoma—Chemotherapy—Evaluation—Congresses.
2. Metipranolol—Testing—Congresses. I. Merté, H.-J. (Hanns-Jürgen). II. Title. RE871.M48. 1983.
617.7'41061. 84-10489.

ISBN 978-3-211-81824-4   ISBN 978-3-7091-4067-3 (eBook)
DOI 10.1007/978-3-7091-4067-3

Dr. Mann Pharma, Berlin, is one of the leading pharmaceutical companies in the field of ophthalmology in the Federal Republic of Germany.

As a result of extensive research and development work a new antiglaucomatous product containing the beta-blocking compound

Metipranolol

was presented in 1982.

This book reports on the results of an international symposium which was held in Berlin in January 1983 to mark the introduction of the new product.

Foreword

After a compound and its various effects — or, as the case may be, any particular one of these — have been discovered there is still a long way ahead until it is available for use in daily practice as a finished product. Before reaching the doctor, the substance is examined by chemists, pharmacologists and pharmacists — just to mention a few of the most important stages in a whole research sequence. Before the drug is finally made available on the market, the findings resulting from animal experiments must be confirmed in clinical studies. The expectations involved in its development must be met, and sufficient evidence has to be established as to the drug's effects and side effects, indications and contraindications, and the questions of safe use and appropriate dosage. Only then may the drug be registered and introduced to the market.

In this respect Metipranolol eye drops, which have recently been launched on the market, formed no exception and had likewise to go through all these various stages. A series of investigators at many different centers participated in this procedure, and at the invitation of the manufacturers, Messrs. Dr. Gerhard Mann, they assembled for discussions at a symposium held in Berlin in January 1983, and reported on the substance and their experiences with it. The contributions seemed so interesting and of such practical importance that it was decided to make them generally available in printed form, and thus this book came into being. In the first section the above-mentioned reports are presented, which in a certain sense form the starting points and the basis for the use of Metipranolol in human studies.

The actual clinical reports — varying in form and purpose — then follow. Thus a good insight into various problems, including those of general significance and not just pertinent to the main issue (Metipranolol eye drops), is provided. The publication of this book may be ascribed on the one hand to the initiative of Messrs. Dr. Mann, on the other hand to the initiative and experience of Springer-Verlag in Vienna. To all persons involved in whatever manner in making this book possible I wish to express my sincere appreciation for their great willingness to help and for their active support at all times.

Munich, April 1983   *H.-J. Merté*

Supplementary Remarks on the English Edition

This book met with great interest and was very readily accepted as it serves to fill a gap in the literature on beta-blocking agents. Nevertheless, the fact that it first appeared in German did seem to be a hindrance to a wider circulation; the request to have the book translated into English, the predominant language in the world of science, was expressed so frequently that both the authors and the publishers felt the need to comply. They now present "Metipranolol — Pharmacology of beta-blocking agents and use of metipranolol in ophthalmology".

I should like to thank those members of the staff of Dr. Mann Pharma and Springer-Verlag who participated in the translating work and printing of this book.

Munich, April 1984   *H.-J. Merté*

Contents

Participants in Symposium

The Chairman:

Prof. Dr. *H.-J. Merté,* Director of the Eye Infirmary and Outpatient Eye Clinic rechts der Isar — Technical University, Munich.

Speakers:

Dr. *W. Bartsch,* Messrs. Boehringer Mannheim GmbH.

Prof. Dr. *H. Bleckmann,* Deputy Director of the University Eye Clinic Charlottenburg, Berlin.

Prof. Dr. *D. Dausch,* Ophthalmologist, Amberg.

Dr. *N. Demmler,* Ophthalmologist, Passau.

Priv. Lecturer Dr. *H. von Denffer,* Assistant Medical Director of the Eye Infirmary and Outpatient Eye Clinic rechts der Isar — Technical University, Munich.

Prof. Dr. *J. Draeger,* Director of the University Eye Clinic and Outpatient Eye Clinic, Hamburg-Eppendorf.

Prof. Dr. *G. K. Krieglstein,* Assistant Medical Director of the University Eye Clinic, Würzburg.

Dr. *W. Kruse,* Ophthalmologist, Berlin.

Priv. Lecturer Dr. *M. Mertz,* Academic Director of the Eye Infirmary and Outpatient Eye Clinic rechts der Isar — Technical University, Munich.

Prof. Dr. *E. Noack,* Pharmacological Institute of the University of Düsseldorf.

Prof. Dr. *D. Palm,* Director of the Center of Pharmacology of the Johann-Wolfgang-Goethe-University, Frankfurt/Main.

Dr. *P. Schmitz-Valckenberg,* Ophthalmologist, Koblenz.

Dr. Dr. *W. Sterner,* IBR Forschungs GmbH, Walsrode.

Dr. *J. Stryz,* Eye Infirmary and Outpatient Eye Clinic rechts der Isar — Technical University, Munich.

Dr. *L. Wawretschek,* Messrs. Dr. Mann Pharma, Berlin.

New Directions in Glaucoma Therapy — Introductory Speech at the Metipranolol Symposium

H.-J. Merté

Eye Infirmary and Outpatient Eye Clinic rechts der Isar —
Technical University, Munich, Federal Republic of Germany

An effective medicamentous glaucoma therapy with its unchanged principle of parasympathomimetic action has been at our disposal for more than 100 years. In the course of the decades there have been additions and modifications to our therapeutic choice of preparations but still those first substances introduced then have asserted their prominent position up to our times. This applies particularly to Pilocarpine. No matter what the principle of action, none of the medicaments introduced since then to reduce pressure has in all these years succeeded in ousting the parasympathomimetic agents in general and Pilocarpine in particular.

It was not until the last ten years that this dominating rôle was challenged by the introduction to ophthalmology of adrenergic beta-receptor blocking agents. A great number of substances of this type is known but their suitability to the given purpose is by no means uniform. This is due to diverse properties and reasons partly of a very varied nature. We, therefore, know some substances which seem more suitable and others which seem less suitable for the treatment of glaucoma, whereby, apart from the pressure reducing effect, a number of typical side effects in particular play a decisive rôle.

As a consequence it was and remains essential to keep looking for optimum substances in order to be able to use these for the benefit of patients. This is why we ophthalmologists are grateful when substances which seem suitable are placed at our disposal so that we can then test their clinical usefulness and investigate their efficiency by means of prolonged usage. Metipranolol is such a substance and it seems particularly promising. We are grateful to

Messrs. Dr. Mann for making it available. This medicament has now been tested in various centres in order to establish the scope of its advantages. The purpose of this symposium today is to give the various investigators an opportunity of exchanging experience and of discussing the results of their tests so that by the end of this day we shall have obtained a certain overall idea of the potential of Metipranolol in glaucoma therapy and be able to provide the ophthalmological profession with a preliminary report on its suitability. Accordingly this symposium fulfils an important function.

Receptor-mediated Effects of Drugs on the Eye

D. Palm

Center of Pharmacology,
Clinic of the Johann-Wolfgang-Goethe University,
Frankfurt/Main, Federal Republic of Germany

With 11 Figures

Innervation and Function, Adrenoceptors and Cholinoceptors

Numerous functions of the eye such as width of pupils, accommodation, possibly also secretion of aqueous humour and the facility of its outflow are regulated almost exclusively via the autonomic nervous system. The dense innervation (for review, see [26]) (for example that of the M. sphincter and M. dilatator pupillae with sympathetic fibers which originate from the ganglion cervicale superius and flow into the muscular effector cells via the Nn. ciliares breves and longi) guarantee a potential release of noradrenaline at the sympathetic nerve endings (Fig. 1). By stimulation of the postsynaptic α_1-adrenoceptors noradrenaline produces a contraction of smooth muscle and, via β-adrenoceptors, a relaxation of smooth muscle.

The parasympathetic cholinergic innervation ensues mainly via the ganglion ciliare and also the ggl. pterygopalatinum via N. oculomotorius. A contraction of smooth muscles is triggered by releasing acetylcholine to the postsynaptic cholinoceptors (Fig. 1). Probably the so-called muscarinic receptors (specific stimulation by the alkaloid muscarine, specific inhibition by atropine) are in the majority whereas the presence of postsynaptic nicotine receptors (specific agonist nicotine, specific antagonist d-tubocurarine) on the inner eye muscles has not so far been clearly demonstrated [22, 26].

Nicotine receptors, however, are the specific cholinoceptors of the outer eye muscles.

A certain selectivity of innervation is obvious in the M. ciliaris: only about 1 % of the detectable autonomic nerve endings are noradrenergic [4]; the cholinergic innervation from the N. oculomotorius prevails whilst a very dense, probably only vascular noradrenergic and cholinergic network can be detected in the processus ciliaris. To what extent neurones, whose neurotransmitter is the "Vasoactive Intestinal Polypeptide" (VIP), are of functional significance has so far not been clearly elucidated [33].

Significance of Receptor Densities

Therefore, in almost all of the functionally important structures of the eye an indication of the prevailing function of noradrenergic or cholinergic neurones is not to be obtained. It is rather the individual density of adrenoceptors or cholinoceptors which determine the main function (e. g. miosis or mydriasis). Furthermore it is known today — at least as far as adrenoceptors are concerned — that not all receptors need to be localized in the direct vicinity of adrenergic synapses. α_2- and β_2-subpopulations are also detectable at effector cells which have not been innervated directly [13]. It has not yet been clearly demonstrated whether these can be stimulated via the plasma catecholamines or whether they do not at all participate in the autonomic regulation and are merely receptors for pharmaceutic agents applied exogenously.

Postsynaptic Receptor Interactions
(see Fig. 1)

The function of the effector cells which is steered noradrenergic-cholinergically and seems to be only two-fold, is supplemented, however, by numerous feed-back mechanisms: it can now be demonstrated postsynaptically that the stimulation of α- and β-adrenoceptors do not only produce pharmaco-dynamically antagonistic effects (i. e. smooth-muscular contraction or relaxation): a mechanism localized in the postsynaptic membrane causes a stimulation of the α_2-adrenoceptors to produce a reduction in the stimulation of the β-adrenoceptor system; also the stimulation of muscarine receptors leads to an inhibition of the β-adrenoceptor system in the postsynaptic membrane [8] (compare Figs. 1, 4, 8).

Presynaptic Feed-back Mechanisms
(see Fig. 1; reports in [13, 29, 30])

Noradrenaline (NA) released from sympathetic nerve endings does not only stimulate postsynaptic α_1-, but also presynaptic α_2-adrenoceptors at noradrenergic and cholinergic nerve endings. NA thus produces an inhibition of its own release and also of that of acetylcholine.

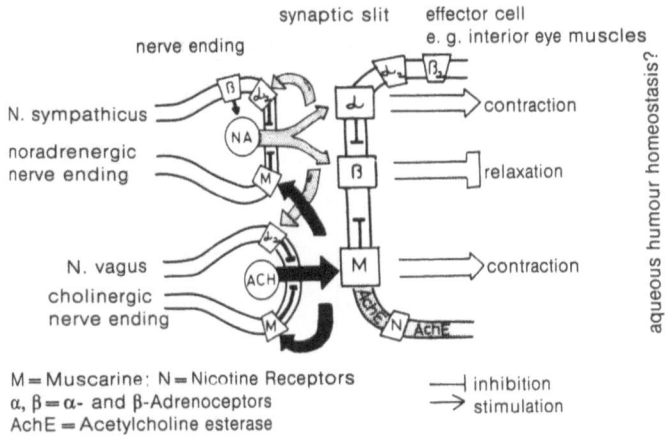

Fig. 1. Pre- and postsynaptic neurotransmitter receptor interactions. Upon the release of noradrenaline and acetylcholine from sympathetic or parasympathetic nerve endings postsynaptic and presynaptic adrenoceptors (α_1, α_2, β_1, β_2) or cholinoreceptors (M, N) can be stimulated. The postsynaptic neurotransmitter receptor interactions trigger the pharmacodynamic effects in the effector organ (but also receptor-receptor interactions: $\alpha \dashv \beta \vdash M$). The presynaptic neurotransmitter receptor interactions bring about negative (or positive) feed-back regulations on the transmitter release. For further details see text (adapted from Greeff and Palm, 1983)

Analogously, acetylcholine inhibits its own release by stimulation of presynaptic muscarine receptors at cholinergic nerve endings and also the release of noradrenaline by stimulation of muscarine receptors at noradrenergic nerve endings. A cholinergic stimulation, therefore, causes an intensified postsynaptic effect (e. g. miosis) by the simultaneous inhibition of the NA release at the M. dilatator pupillae. The mydriatic "sympathomimetic" action (for example of atropine, a specific inhibitor of acetylcholine at muscarine receptors) is therefore produced not only via an inhibition of the postsynaptic muscarine receptors at the M. sphincter pupillae but also by an intensified release of NA to the M. dilatator pupillae by inhibition of presynaptic muscarine receptors at noradrenergic nerve endings (cf. Fig. 1).

Receptor-specific Effects of Drugs

By means of chemical modification of neurotransmitters the attempt was made to develop receptor-specific drugs which could imitate the effect of a sympathetic-noradrenergic or parasympathetic-cholinergic stimulus of the nerve and also demonstrate certain receptor selectivities (Fig. 2).

Adrenoceptors		Cholinoceptors
α	β	M
Noradrenaline		Acetylcholine
Adrenaline		Carbachol (2)
Phenylephrine		N - Desmethyl - Carbachol
Clonidine	Isoprenaline	Pilocarpine
Naphazoline	Fenoterol	Physostigmine
Xylometazoline	Salbutamol	Neostigmine [2]
Tetryzoline	Terbutaline	DFP
Tyramine [1]		Ecothiopate [3]

[1] indirectly active   [2] Reversible and   [3] Irreversible inhibitors of acetylcholine esterase

Fig. 2. Agonists at α- and β-adrenoceptors (α, β) as well as at cholinoceptors (muscarine receptors, M) of the internal ocular muscles (incomplete selection). The receptor specificity can be demonstrated by receptor blockers (α-receptor blockers: phentolamine; β-receptor blockers: propranolol; muscarine receptor blockers: atropine)

As well as the α- and β-sympathomimetically active catecholamines adrenaline and noradrenaline the mainly α-sympathomimetic active derivative phenylephrine and the imidazoline derivatives clonidine, naphazoline etc. have been used as topical ophthalmic preparations to produce a mydriasis or vasoconstriction. Their action is — under experimental conditions — inhibited by the α-receptor blocking agents phentolamine and prazosine.

Isoprenaline and its derivatives, which act mainly on β_2-adreno-ceptors (fenoterol etc.), were used for test purposes to reduce increased intraocular pressure. Agonists on muscarine receptors (miotic agents, antiglaucomatous agents) are more lipophil and, as opposed to the inactivating effect of acetylcholine esterase, more stable derivatives of acetylcholine (e. g. pilocarpine). In future more significicance might be attached to the N-demethylated derivative of carbachol* as it is said to have strong antiglaucomatous effects without marked undesired effects such as miosis, disorders of accommodation, reduction of heart frequency etc. [2]. Tyramine is an indirect sympathomimetic agent, not active at receptors. It releases noradrenaline. The indirectly active parasympathomimetic agents are inhibitors of acetylcholine esterase. The endogenous acetylcholine concentration active at muscarine receptors is increased over a long period; the receptor stimulation is intensified. All cholinergic effects are inhibited specifically by the muscarine receptor blocking agent (= parasympatholytic) atropine.

Receptor Specificity, Intensity and Organ Selectivity of Actions Mediated by Receptors

Originally receptors could only be defined operationally on the basis of the pharmacodynamic effects produced by their stimulation. These had to be inhibited competitively and reversibly by receptor-specific antagonists (receptor blocking agents). Nowadays neurotransmitter receptors are describable as units of the cytoplasmic membrane and can be detected biochemically and quantitatively by means of selective radioactive ligands (for review, see [14]). Receptors are directed against the extracellular space and they recognize and bind neurotransmitters or similar derivatives contained in the synaptic cleft with high affinity corresponding to their chemical constitutional characteristics. This stimulus triggers off a cascade of biochemical reactions, e. g. coupling with an enzyme directed against the intracellular space. The activation of this enzyme produces a cascade of metabolic events which finally leads to enzyme activations with metabolic effects as well as an opening or closing of ion channels in the cytoplasmic membrane; an increase in the Ca^{2+} flux from the extracellular into the intracellular space, mediated by α-adrenoceptors results in smooth muscular contrac-

---

* Carbachol is a stimulator of muscarine receptors and reversibly inhibits acetylcholine esterase; cf. Fig. 2: (2).

tion, e. g. of the M. dilatator pupillae (Fig. 4). Basically the same
pharmacodynamic effect can be produced by a stimulation of muscarine receptors: also the cholinergic depolarisation (Na^+ influx)
increases the Ca^{2+} influx whereby above all the contractions of the
M. sphincter pupillae and the M. ciliaris are triggered off. Vice
versa, one has to reckon with a smooth-muscular relaxation upon

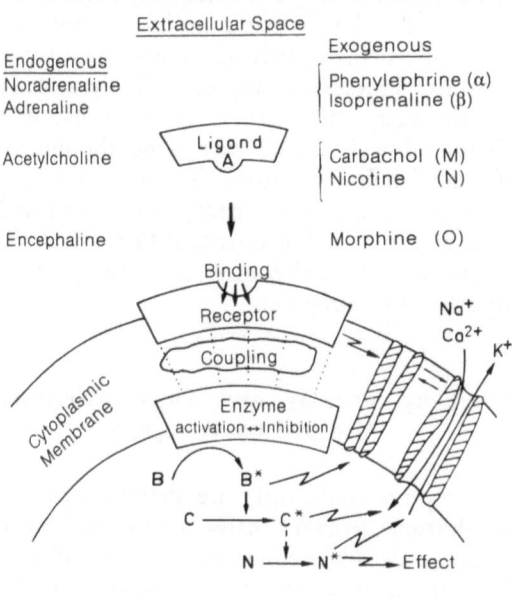

Fig. 3. Schematic illustration of neurotransmitter receptor interaction and
the subsequent stimulation of effector systems. Upon recognition and binding of the agonist present in the extracellular space the receptor stimulation is transmitted to the intracellular space by activation or inhibition of
an enzyme: a) via biochemical cascade of reaction, b) by direct opening or
closing of ion channels. Also receptor antagonists (receptor blocking
agents) are recognized and bound. Subsequent effector systems are not
activated. Antagonists bound with high affinity block the binding of
agonists! (See also Fig. 8)

stimulation of β-adrenoceptors on account of an inhibition of the
Ca^{2+} influx (slighter Ca^{2+} channel width, lower number of open
channels) (Fig. 4).

The receptor is thus decisive for the selectivity of a pharmacological effect: on the basis of the specific capacity to recognize cer-

tain chemical configurations and on the basis of the effector systems coupled to the receptors. The cascade of reactions adopts the function of an amplifier. Because of this 1 drug molecule (agonist) can induce up to 10^6 effector molecules (N*; Fig. 3).

The receptor density is decisive for the organ selectivity of the effect.

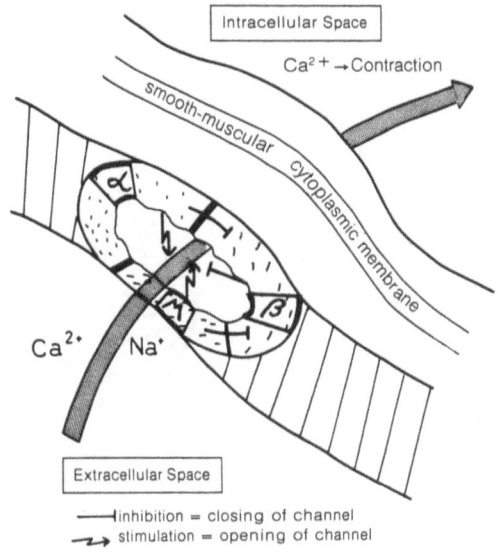

Fig. 4. Schematic illustration of receptor-mediated effects (Ion permeabilities). By stimulation of α-adrenoceptors (α) or muscarine receptors (M) the calcium permeability increase (↗): the increase of the calcium concentration in the intracellular space produces smooth-muscular contraction. A β-sympathomimetic inhibition of Ca^{2+} influx triggers off a smooth-muscular relaxation. Stimulation of M- and α-receptors causes postsynaptic inhibition (⊣) of β-adrenoceptors. (Compare Fig. 1)

Cholinergic effects on muscarine receptors dominate wherever there is a preponderance of muscarine receptors (Glandula lacrimalis, M. ciliaris, M. sphincter pupillae) (Fig. 5). The muscarine receptor blocking agent atropine, therefore — apart from its mydriatic effect (paralysis of the M. sphincter pupillae) — cannot fail but to produce an inhibition of the secretion of the lacrimal gland and a paralysis of the M. ciliaris with subsequent paralysis of accommodation and, in certain circumstances, reduction of the facility of aqueous outflow. In contrast to this the α_1-adrenergically produced mydriasis (contraction of the M. dilatator pupillae) is of necessity free from such undesired effects.

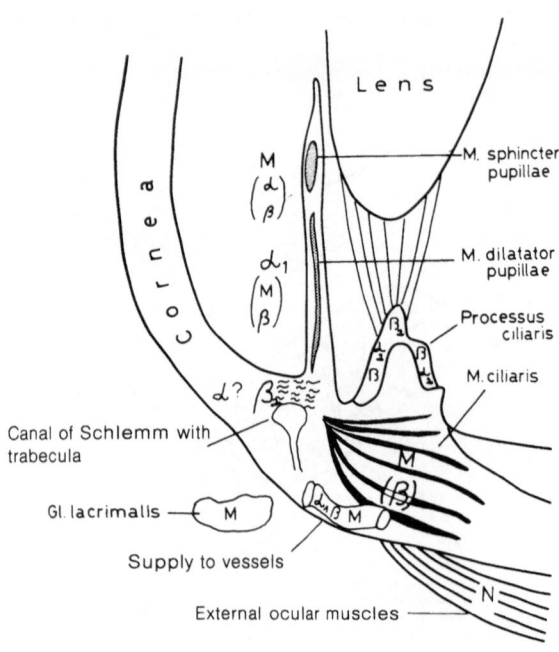

Fig. 5

	Regulation of tonus of the inner ocular muscles		
	M. sphincter p.	M. dilatator p.	M. ciliaris
Muscarine Receptors	+ + + + ⬆	+ + Presynaptic? ⇓	+ + + + ⬆
α-Adreno-ceptors	+ + Presynaptic? ⇓	+ + + + ⬆	(+) ⇑
β-Adreno-ceptors	+ ⇩	+ ⇩	+ + + ⇩
Atropine effect	⬇⬇⬇ Mydriasis	⬆⬆	⬇ accommodation paralysis

Fig. 6

A more detailed pharmacodynamic analysis of the adrenoceptors and cholinoceptors of the internal smooth ocular muscle shows, however, (Figs. 5 and 6) that all 3 muscles are equipped with 3 types of receptors [9]. The dominating receptor population, however, determines the therapeutically relevant effect (or side effect).

Corresponding to the illustration the mydriatic effect of atropine is as follows: inhibition of the cholinergic contraction of the M. sphincter pupillae, inhibition of the cholinergic relaxation of the M. dilatator pupillae with persisting or even intensified α-adrenergic contracting effect on the M. dilatator pupillae; furthermore there are dilating α- and β-adrenergic effects on the M. sphincter pupillae (Fig. 6).

Effects of Drugs on the Homeostasis of the Aqueous Humour
(Reviews in [2, 24, 25])

Receptor-mediated effects of drugs on the homeostasis of the aqueous humour are much more complex and in the main with regard to their individual mechnisms unclarified and contradictory.

In many cases the effect of drugs are describable or definable only on the basis of purely empirical methods for the intraocular pressure is regulated by the manifold interaction of numerous processes. In simple words, however, it may be said that the homeostasis of intraocular pressure is primarily determined by the formation of aqueous humour (ultrafiltration, secretion) and the outflow of aqueous humour (Fig. 7).

Drugs which in the main decrease intraocular pressure by increasing the facility of outflow are agonists at muscarine receptors (e. g. pilocarpine) (for review, see [10]) as well as the agonists at the α- and β-adrenoceptors adrenaline and noradrenaline [27, 28].

Fig. 5. Dominating receptor distributions on the eye. Functionally unimportant receptors in brackets. M muscarine receptors; N nicotine receptors (on the outer ocular muscles); α and β adrenoceptors

Fig. 6. Receptor-mediated contraction ($\uparrow$) or relaxation ($\downarrow$) of the inner ocular muscles. The "receptor densities" obtained from pharmacodynamic studies are marked from + up to + + + (according to results by Kern [9]). The paradoxical relaxation of the M. sphincter pupillae mediated via α-adrenoceptors is possibly of a presynaptic nature (inhibition of the release of acetylcholine); this may probably be similarly relevant for the relaxing effect of acetylcholine on the M. dilatator pupillae (inhibition of release of noradrenaline. (Compare Fig. 1)

Via a stimulation of muscarine receptors (atropine is a specific receptor antagonist) pilocarpine and other muscarine receptor stimulants produce a stretching and unfurling of the trabecula lamellae placed before the Schlemm's canal. A widening of the passages of flow and thus an increase in the facility of outflow results from

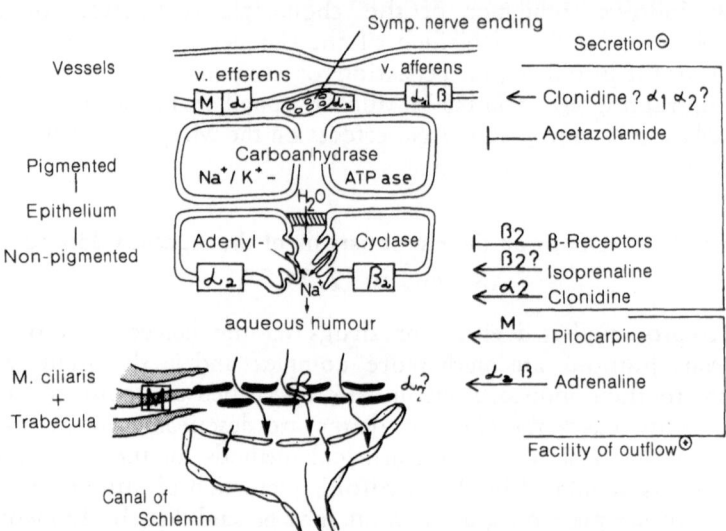

Fig. 7. Schematic illustration of the mechanisms of the formation and outflow of aqueous humour. Localization of receptors and enzymes which could illustrate the sites of action of drugs with effect on formation of aqueous humour and/or facility of outflow

a widening of the cribiform region [16]. Miotic and undesired effects changing accommodation are necessarily involved in this undesired action.

In contrast to this the mechanism of the intraocular pressure lowering effect of adrenaline and noradrenaline is hypothetical to a great extent, for the direct proof of α-adrenoceptors in the range of the trabecular meshwork has still to be given. β-adrenoceptors could so far only be identified in cultivated human trabecula cells [1].

Sears postulates [27, 28]: in the initial phase adrenaline reduces ultrafiltration of the aqueous humour by α_1-adrenergic vasoconstriction of the vasa afferentia in the ciliary body. At the same time an α-adrenergic (α_2?) increase in outflow facility occurs. For the intermediary main effect a β-adrenergically increased cAMP formation in the endothelial cells of Schlemm's canal is postulated. As a β-sympathomimetic delayed action after long-term administration a change in the glucosaminoglucanes of the trabecular meshwork is said to bring about an increase of the facility of outflow.

Aqueous humour formation on the basis of an ultrafiltration is dependent on the pressure of arterial perfusion. It is reasonable

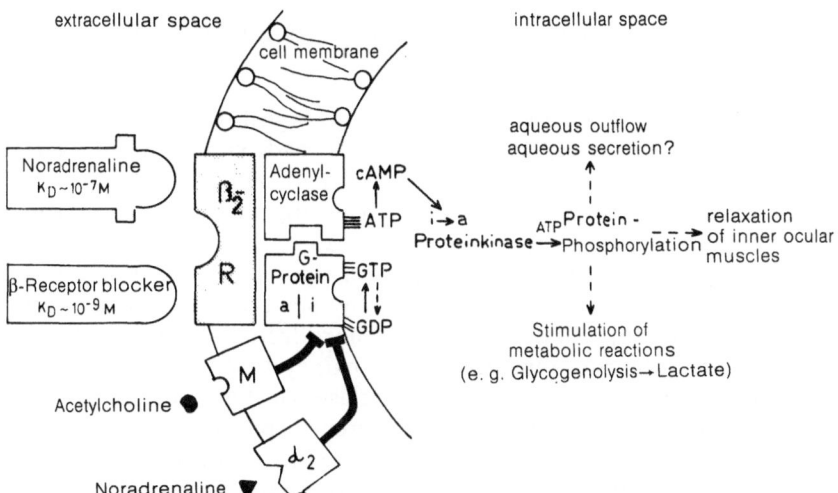

Fig. 8. Schematic illustration of β-adrenoceptors and the after-connected effector systems (with pharmacodynamical and biochemical effects on the eye). The β-adrenoceptor stimulation by agonists leads via the coupling β-adrenoceptor → active subunit of the guanylnucleotide binding proteins → adenylcyclase to an increased formation of cAMP in the intracellular space. By this β-sympathomimetic pharmacodynamic reactions are triggered off via an enzymatic cascade of reactions. It has so far not been clarified why stimulation and blockade of β-adrenoceptors produce an inhibition in the production of aqueous humour

that an α_1-adrenergic vasoconstriction, e. g. by clonidine, can produce a reduction in intraocular pressure. However, other sites of action must also be made valid for the effect of clonidine, e. g. inhibition of the noradrenaline release by stimulation of central or peripheral α_2-adrenoceptors. Clonidine could also inhibit β_2-adrenoceptors via the stimulation of α_2-adrenoceptors [5—7] (Figs. 7 and 8).

The activities of Na^+-K^+-ATP and of carbonic anhydrase in epithelial cells of the ciliary appendix seem to be of essential significance for the aqueous humour secretion; they provide the prerequisite for the aqueous penetration through the zonulae occludentes (blood aqueous barrier) at the basis of the non-pigmented epithelial cells; it is the ionic gradient which induces a passive water diffusion [16].

It is reasonable that an inhibition of the carbonic anhydrase by acetazolamide therefore limits the process of secretion aculety.

β_2-Adrenoceptor Agonists and Antagonists as Inhibitors of Aqueous Secretion

In which way β-receptor agonists and antagonists inhibit aqueous secretion is completely unclear — and paradoxical! On the basis of numerous findings it has been clearly established that a high density of β-adrenoceptors is localized in the epithelial cell of the ciliary body [19, 21] (for review, see [24, 25]).

All findings hitherto indicate the existence of β_2-adrenoceptors and this can be proven with relatively selective β_2-agonists and β_2-antagonists [6]. The fact that no noradrenergic nerve endings can be proven in the epithelium of the ciliary body is in conformity with this [26]. There is an adenylcyclase of high activity in the ciliary body post-connected to the β_2-adrenoceptors [18] (for review, see [24 and 25]). This is the effector enzyme which upon stimulation of the β-adrenoceptor unit directed against the extracellular space (e. g. by the physiological agonist noradrenaline) transmits the extracellular stimulus to the intracellular space (Fig. 8). Via a biochemical cascade of reactions the increased cAMP formation produces the stimulation of metabolic reactions and a smooth-muscular relaxation. The mechanism of the facilitation of aqueous outflow induced by cAMP is unclear [19]. That cAMP also promotes aqueous secretion can only be deduced from the fact that all β-receptor blocking agents reduce aqueous secretion and thus intraocular pressure; therefore, it seems paradoxical that isoproterenol and a series of β_2-sympathomimetic agents likewise reduce aqueous secretion and thus intraocular pressure [31] (for review, see [24 and 25]). The fact that the stimulation success at the β-adrenoceptors can be switched off by stimulation of muscarine receptors or α_2-adrenoceptors speaks for the multitude of vegetative regulatory mechanisms (Fig. 8).

β-receptor blockers bind to the β-adrenoceptors with a 100 to 1000-fold higher affinity than β-receptor agonists; however — contrary to β-adrenoceptor agonists — they do not trigger off any coupling between β-adrenoceptor, G-protein und adenylcyclase and thus they do not cause any subsequent reactions: receptor blockers are drugs with high affinity and without intrinsic activity. Due to their high affinity, however, the endogenous agonist is competitively displaced from the receptor, the receptor is blocked reversibly. The "blockade" can, however, be interrupted competitively by higher agonist concentrations.

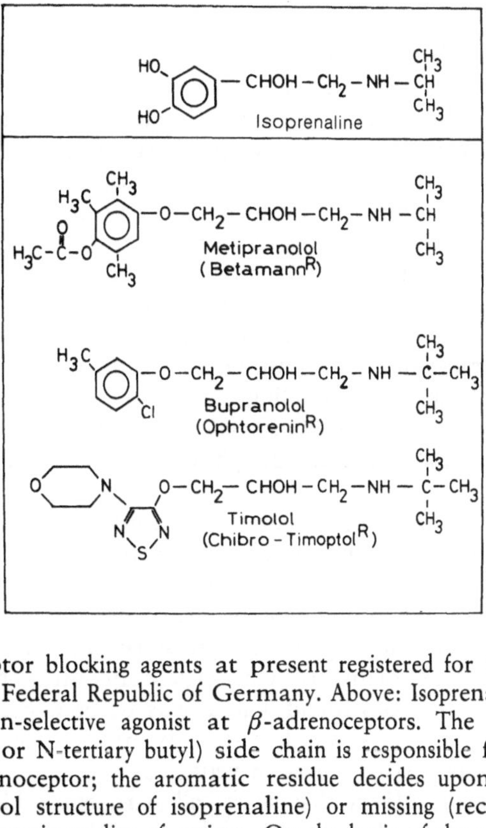

Fig. 9. β-receptor blocking agents at present registered for topical use on the eye in the Federal Republic of Germany. Above: Isoprenaline as proto-type of a non-selective agonist at β-adrenoceptors. The ethanolamine-(N-isopropyl- or N-tertiary butyl) side chain is responsible for the affinity to the β-adrenoceptor; the aromatic residue decides upon available in-trinsic (catechol structure of isoprenaline) or missing (receptor blocker) β sympathomimetic quality of action. On the basis of the optically active center at the $-$CHOH group there are ($-$)-enantiomers of 100-fold higher affinity than ($+$)-enantiomers. The aromatic residue is decisive for the physico-chemical property "lipophilicity"

It may be stated in favour of a specific reduction of intraocular pressure triggered off by a β-receptor blockade that *all* β-receptor blocking agents tested so far possess this desired action upon topi-cal, parenteral or oral application — understandably without un-desired effects on width of pupils, lacrimal secretion or accommodation [12]. At the moment metipranolol, bupranolol and timolol are commercialized in the Federal Republic of Germany for the topical treatment of "Glaucoma". Compared to the β-adrenoceptor agonist isoprenaline these demonstrate the typical chemical constitutional property of β-receptor antagonists (Fig. 9).

On the basis of present model ideas about the dynamics of receptor-effector systems [15, 17, 32] it can be deduced that a chronic stimulation of the receptor produces a densensitization, a reduction in the receptor density and thus, under certain circumstances, also a decrease in the beta-sympathomimetic action. A "desensitization", however, can also occur when the density of the receptor units increases due to a chronically weakened stimulation of the receptor or a chronic blockade by receptor. It should, however, be possible to interrupt this tolerance by increasing the concentration of the antagonist. In fact the "antiglaucomatous effect" of timolol which decreases in sub-chronic and chronic application suggests such a tolerance [11, 12. 24]. It has not been clarified to what extent an increase of the receptor units can be made responsible for a weakening of the therapeutic effect [30]. Other "weak points" of the receptor effector system (e. g. coupling unit = G-protein between receptor and adenylcyclase as well as single stages in the effector cascade) could also be responsible for the phenomenon of tolerance [15, 17] (see Fig. 8).

The objection has been made that timolol would trigger off its intraocular pressure reducing effect via non-specific effects not dependent on β-adrenoceptors (e. g. inhibition of Na^+-K^+-ATP in the ciliary epithelial membrane by hydrophobic interactions); for (+)- and (−)-Timolol apparently prove to have the same strong effect in animal experiments (with high concentrations) [2]. However, other investigators found that, as was to be expected, the effect of the (+)-enantiomers was less strongly marked than that of the (−)-enantiomers [3]. It may nevertheless be said on behalf of a receptor-specific effect that so far all β-receptor blocking agents have been able to reduce increased or normal intraocular pressure to matter what the form of application.

The hypothetical example of figures given in Fig. 10 shows that, both under experimental and therapeutical conditions, the (+)-enantiomer which possesses $1/100$ of the β-blocking affinity of the (−)-enantiomer can exert an effective β-receptor blocking effect: even on the assumption that only 1 per cent of the applied drug quantity becomes effective on homogeneous distribution the 100-fold weaker affinity of (+)-metipranolol suffices to inhibit the β-adrenoceptors of the ciliary epithelium by 50%.

A further objection to a receptor-specific action of β-receptor-blockers in the treatment of glaucoma is the following: the effect is of long duration; topical application 1—2 times daily is sufficient to lower intraocular pressure constantly.

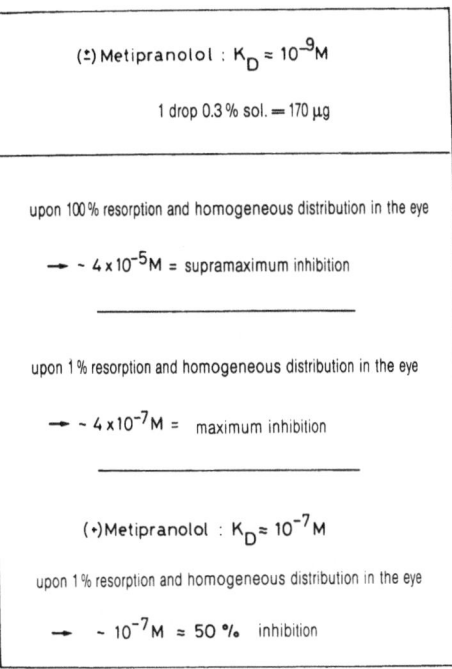

Fig. 10. Metipranolol concentration upon topical application and predictable inhibitory action on β-adrenoceptors on the eye. Hypothetical calculation example (see: prerequisites). K_D molar concentration which is necessary for 50% inhibition of the receptor

The assisting hypothesis that on the basis of hydrophobic interactions pigmented epithelia represent a β-receptor blocker depot which slowly liberates the active ingredient [21] may well be true but it seems to be decisive that the half life period (e. g. in the plasma for Metipranolol ~ 3 hours) and half period of the pharmacodynamic action are bound via the equation "Pharmacological Effect" $= K_i \cdot \log$ concentration $+ K_2$. As can be seen from Fig. 11, the active concentration is reduced by 50 per cent within 3 hours, whereas a maximal inhibitory effect on the half-maximum action does not decrease until after 6—9 hours.

On the basis of Fig. 11 it can be assumed that initially supramaximum active concentrations are present in the eye so that e. g.
after 9 hours there should still be a 100% inhibition of β-adreno-

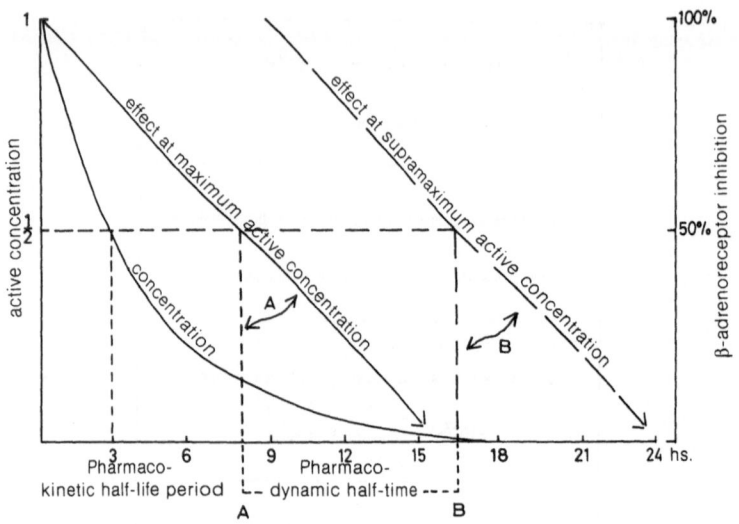

Fig. 11. Extent of a β-adrenoceptor blockade (right ordinate) in relation to
local concentration (left ordinate) and time (abscissa). The active concentration decreases according to a reaction of the 1st order. The effect
decreases almost according to a reaction of 0 order. After 100% adreno-
ceptor inhibition and a kinetic half-life period of approx. 3 hours a half-
maximum inhibition is still to be reckoned with after 6—9 hours. If the
active concentration is supramaximal (compare Fig. 10) e. g. for the duration of 9 hours there is a 100% blockade of the receptor for 9 hours.
Correspondingly, a half-maximum drug action is not to be expected until
after 15—18 hours. Apparently the pharmacological effect decreases more
slowly than corresponds to the decrease in active concentration. The effect
is almost proportional to the logarithm of the concentration!
A Pharmacodynamical half-time at initially maximum inhibitory concentration $(1 \to 100\%)$. B Pharmacodynamic half-time at supramaximum inhibitory concentration $(\gg 1)$

ceptors which only decreases to a half-maximum inhibitory effect
in the course of further 6—9 hours. So far, however, exact data
about the intraocular pharmacokinetics of β-receptor blockers are
not available.

References

1. Bloom, E., Polansky, J., Zlock, D., Wood, I., Alvarado, J., Zumbrum, A.: Timolol and epinephrine binding to isolated ciliary epithelium and trabecular cells. Invest. Ophthalmol. Visual. Sci. (A. R. V. O.) 20, 66 (1981).

2. Chiou, G. C. Y.: Recent advances in antiglaucoma drugs. Biochem. Pharmacol. 30, 103—106 (1981).

3. Colosanti, B. K., Trotter, R. R.: Effects of selective beta$_1$- and beta$_2$-adrenoceptor agonists and antagonists on intraocular pressure in the cat. Invest. Ophthalmol. Visual Sci. 20, 69—76 (1981).

4. Ehinger, B.: A comparative study of the adrenergic nerves to the anterior eye segment of some primates. Z. Zellforsch. 116, 157—177 (1971).

5. Innemee, H. C., van Zwieten, P. A.: The central nervous influence of drugs on intraocular pressure. Rev. Pure and Appl. Pharmacol. Sci. 1, 107—165 (1980).

6. Innemee, H. C., de Jonge, A., van Meel, J. C. A., Timmermanns, P. B. M. W. M., van Zwieten, P. A.: The effect of selective α_1 and α_2-adrenoceptor stimulation on intraocular pressure in the conscious rabbit. Naunyn-Schmiedebergs Arch. Pharmacol. 316, 294—298 (1981).

7. Innemee, H. C., van Zwieten, P. A.: The role of β_2-adrenoceptors in the IOP-lowering effect of adrenaline. Graefes Arch. Klin. Exp. Ophthalmol. 218, 297—300 (1982).

8. Jakobs, K. H., Aktories, K., Schultz, G.: Inhibition of adenylate cyclase by hormones and neurotransmitters. Adv. Cycl. Nucl. Res. 14, 173—187 (1981).

9. Kern, R.: Die adrenergischen Rezeptoren der intraoculären Muskeln des Menschen. Eine In-vitro-Studie. Graefes Arch. Klin. Exp. Ophthalmol. 180, 231—248 (1970).

10. Krieglstein, G. K.: Pharmakologische Grundlagen der Therapie mit Miotika. Klin. Monatsbl. Augenheilk. 163, 471—476 (1973).

11. Krieglstein, G. K.: Die Wirkung von Timolol-Augentropfen auf den Augeninnendruck bei Glaukoma simplex. Klin. Monatsbl. Augenheilk. 172, 677—685 (1978).

12. Krieglstein, G. K.: Betablockertherapie der Glaukome. In: Medikamentöse Glaukomtherapie (Krieglstein, G. K., Leydhecker, W., eds.), pp. 29—40. München: Bergmann. 1982.

13. Langer, S. Z.: Presynaptic regulation of the release of catecholamines. Pharmacol. Rev. 32, 337—362 (1981).

14. Lamble, J. W. (ed.): More About Receptors (Current Rev. Biomed., Vol. 2). Amsterdam—New York—Oxford: Elsevier Biomedical Press. 1982.

15. Lefkowitz, R. J.: Clinical physiology of adrenergic receptor regulation. Am. J. Physiol. 243, E. 43—47 (1982).

16. Lütjen-Drecoll, E.: Morphologische Grundlagen der Glaukomtherapie. In: Medikamentöse Glaukomtherapie (Krieglstein, G. K., Leydhecker, W., eds.), pp. 3—11. München: Bergmann. 1982.

17. Motulsky, H. J., Insel, P. A.: Adrenergic receptors in man. Direct identification, physiologic regulation und clinical alterations. New. Engl. J. Med. 307, 18—29 (1982).

18. Nathanson, J. A.: Adrenergic regulation of intraocular pressure: Identification of β_2-adrenergic-stimulated adenylate cyclase in ciliary process epithelium. Proc. Natl. Acad. Sci. (U. S. A.) 77, 7420—7424 (1980).

19. Neufeld, A. H.: Influences of cyclic nucleotides on outflow facility in the vervet monkey. Exp. Eye Res. 27, 387—397 (1978).

20. Neufeld, A. H., Zawistowski, K. A., Page, E. D., Bromberg, B. B.: Influence on the density of β-adrenergic receptors in the cornea and iris-ciliary body of the rabbit. Invest. Ophthalmol. Visual Sci. 17, 1069—1075 (1978).

21. Neufeld, A. H., Bartels, S. P.: Receptor mechanisms for epinephrine and timolol. In: Basic Aspects of Glaucoma Research (Lütjen-Drecoll, E., ed.), pp. 113—122. Stuttgart—New York: Schattauer. 1982.

22. Nilsson, J., Linder, J., Bill, A.: Effects of facial nerve stimulation on ocular blood flow and the intraocular pressure (IOP) in the cynomolgus monkey. Acta Physiol. Scand. 109, D 18 (1980).

23. Philipps, C. I., Howitt, G., Rowland, D. J.: Propranolol as ocular hypotensive agent. Brit. J. Ophthalmol. 51, 222—226 (1967).

24. Potter, D. E.: Adrenergic pharmacology of aqueous humor dynamics. Pharmacol. Rev. 33, 133—153 (1981).

25. Potter, D. E., Rowland, J. M.: Adrenergic drugs and intraocular pressure. Gen. Pharmacol. 12, 1—13 (1981).

26. Ruskell, G. L.: Innervation of the anterior segment of the eye. In: Basic Aspects of Glaucoma Research (Lütjen-Drecoll, E., ed.), pp. 49—66. Stuttgart—New York: Schattauer. 1982.

27. Sears, M. L.: Perspectives in the medical treatment of glaucoma. In: Medikamentöse Glaukomtherapie (Krieglstein, G. K., Leydhecker, W., eds.), pp. 49—58. München: Bergmann. 1982.

28. Sears, M. L., Neufeld, A. H.: Adrenergic modulation of the outflow of aqueous humor. Invest. Ophthalmol. 14, 83—86 (1975).

29. Starke, K.: Regulation of noradrenaline release by presynaptic receptor systems. Rev. Physiol. Biochem. Pharmacol. 77, 1—124 (1977).

30. Starke, K.: Presynaptic receptors. Ann. Rev. Pharmacol. Toxicol. 21, 7—30 (1981).

31. Thomas, J. V.: Ocular adrenergic receptor sites pertinent to aqueous humor dynamics. Ann. Ophthalmol. 12, 96—98 (1980).

32. Trendelenburg, U.: Über- und Unterempfindlichkeit autonom innervierter Organe. In: Medikamentöse Glaukomtherapie (Krieglstein, G. K., Leydhecker, W., eds.), pp. 19—28. München: Bergmann. 1982.

33. Uddman, R., Alumets, J., Ehinger, B., Håkanson, R., Lorén, I., Sundler, F.: Vasoactive intestinal peptide nerves in ocular and orbital structures of the cat. Invest. Ophthalmol. Visual. Sci. *19*, 878—885 (1980).

Author's address: Prof. Dr. D. Palm, Zentrum der Pharmakologie, Klinikum der Johann-Wolfgang-Goethe-Universität, Theodor-Stern-Kai 7, D-6000 Frankfurt/Main, Federal Republic of Germany.

Present Day Possibilities of Glaucoma Therapy

H.-J. Merté and **J. Stryz**

Eye Infirmary and Outpatient Clinic rechts der Isar —
Technical University, Munich
(Director: Prof. Dr. med. H.-J. Merté),
Federal Republic of Germany

With 15 Figures

If the following succeeds in giving a brief outline of present day possibilities of treating glaucomas with drugs, the aim is to provide an introductory basis to the clinical part dealing with the main issue of the symposium, a synopsis of which is now presented in this book. Even although most doctors will be familiar with the problems from their everyday experience, this summary is intended to accentuate the specific possibilities of the substance dealt with in the following papers and to illustrate clearly the position it occupies in the system of therapy.

Common to the pathogenetic, in part very diverse diseases which are classified in this group and designated as glaucoma, is damage of the optic nerve fibers in the papilla region due to an influence of intraocular pressure, whatever the type may be. The two main elements involved are the pressure tolerance of the optic nerve fibers on the one hand and the level of the intraocular tension on the other (Fig. 1). If the optic nerve fibers are very resistant a considerable increase in pressure is required to cause damage. There may, therefore, be eyes which demonstrate — also for a prolonged period — a pressure above the statistical range, without any damage to the optic nerve fibers being perceptible. In such cases it has become common practice to speak of ocular hypertension. This is the one extreme.

If the resistance of the optic nerve to the consequences of a pressure effect is reduced, in some circumstances an ocular pressure which is within the statistical range of normal and may even be relatively low can also lead to damage typical of glaucoma. In such cases one speaks of glaucoma without high pressure. That is the other extreme.

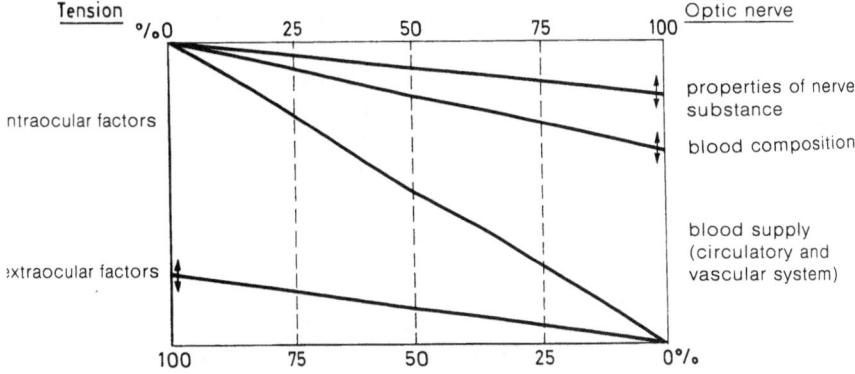

Fig. 1. Factors of damage to optic nerve

In the great majority of cases both components are most likely involved in the development and, above all, the progression of these sequelae.

From this it may be concluded that any increase in the power of resistance of the optic nerve fibers due to an improvement in blood circulation can represent an important therapeutic factor. These reflections, however, should not be pursued at this point, as these problems cannot be resolved by the ophthalmologist on his own anyway, but require cooperation with an internist who is experienced in cardiovascular matters. Nevertheless in this area also one should in some individual cases endeavour to go about the matter in the manner which seems most appropriate for the case in question.

As has ever been the case, pathologically increased intraocular pressure can best be influenced by therapeutic measures. There is no point in elaborating further on the causes of glaucoma here but it must be mentioned that in certain circumstances the pathogenic mechanisms of glaucomas which vary from one another also require various therapeutic measures. Every glaucoma does not respond in the same manner to the given therapeutic possibilities. Quite generally, however, it can be said that chronic glaucomas

are, if possible, to be treated conservatively and only when a very
accurate diagnosis has been made should an operation be carried
out.

Nowadays a great number of drugs are available for the conserv-
ative treatment of glaucomas. Quite generally one can differentiate
between drug effects which are directed at increasing aqueous
outflow on the one hand and limiting the formation of aqueous
humour on the other. Nevertheless it must be borne in mind that
most of the drugs commonly used are not only able to produce the
one effect or the other alone but are frequently, even if to a very
different extent, able to bring about both.

This is also why it is so important to carry out tension adjust-
ments individually in each case and to achieve the optimum result
by testing. In this connection it must be mentioned that combinations of substances with various sites of action occasionally prove
to be more suitable than single-entity drugs. Besides, if chosen right-
ly, they offer the advantage that the undesired side effects of individual ingredients can be kept to a relatively low level with a maximum pressure reducing effect. The most important principles of
drugs commonly used today in glaucoma therapy to reduce pressure
are: substances influencing the peripheral vegetative nervous system,
carbonic anhydrase inhibiting substances, osmotically effective substances and drugs acting via the central nerval system (Fig. 2).

Reduction in intraocular pressure by

1. Influencing the vegetative nervous system or its receptors.
2. Carbonic anhydrase inhibition.
3. Osmotherapy.
4. Central action.

Fig. 2. Possibilities of reducing ocular pressure

The first group in particular is of significance in maintenance
therapy. Drugs of the fourth group can be administered additionally
in some cases. Osmotherapy is indicated solely for short-term reduction of intraocular pressure and may not be repeated constantly.
Carbonic anhydrase inhibitors are sometimes described for a prolonged period but this is, if at all possible, to be avoided on account
of a series of very undesirable side effects affecting the entire organism.

With regard to those substances with an onset of action at the
automatic nervous system one must differentiate between four main

groups (Fig. 3): the parasympathomimetics, the sympathomimetics, the parasympatholytics and the sympatholytics.

In the group of parasympatholytics, e. g. Atropine, the pressure increasing component mostly stands to the fore. Except in certain secondary glaucomas usage to decrease tension can only be considered in very special exceptions, particularly for a short time in a congenital glaucoma during earliest infancy.

Reduction of ocular pressure by

Sympathomimetics   —   Parasympatholytics

Parasympathomimetics —   Sympatholytics

Fig. 3. Possibilities of reducing ocular pressure by influencing the vegetative nervous system

Parasympathomimetics still form the most important group. Here we have to differentiate between the direct and indirect parasympathomimetics, according to the mode of action (Fig. 4).

Direct Parasympathomimetics (Cholinergics)	Indirect Parasympathomimetics (Anticholinesterases)
Acetylcholine	Reversible anticholinesterases
Metacholine	Physostigmine (Eserine)
Pilocarpine	Neostigmine (Prostigmine)
Aceclidine (Glaucotat)	Pyridostigmine (Mestinon)
Carbachol	Distigmine bromide (Ubretide)
	Demecarium bromide (Tosmilene)
	Irreversible anticholinesterases
	Fluostigmine (DFP)
	Paraoxone (Mintacol)
	Echothiophate (Phospholine iodide)

Fig. 4. Direct and indirect parasympathomimetics (selection).
(Quoted from Heilmann)

Indirect in this sense means that the drug inhibits the enzyme (cholinesterase) which degrades the natural parasympathetic transmitting substance (acetylcholine) so that a considerable quantity of acetylcholine is present at the receptor.

Normally the indirect parasympathomimetics are stronger in action than the direct. This is particularly so with regard to substances inhibiting the cholinesterase irreversibly whereas a reversible inhibition of the enzyme activity abates after a somewhat short period. The stronger action of the parasympathomimetics is, the stronger the undesired side effects prove to be. In the long run irreversibly inhibiting substances proved to be so damaging that, if possible, they should not be used at all — at least not for prolonged periods.

Sympathomimetics i. e. substances which produce an increase in adrenergic effects, generally cause a vasoconstriction. Thus their usage is involved with the potential risk of influencing the blood supply of the retina negatively and possibly also that of the optic nerve (Fig. 5).

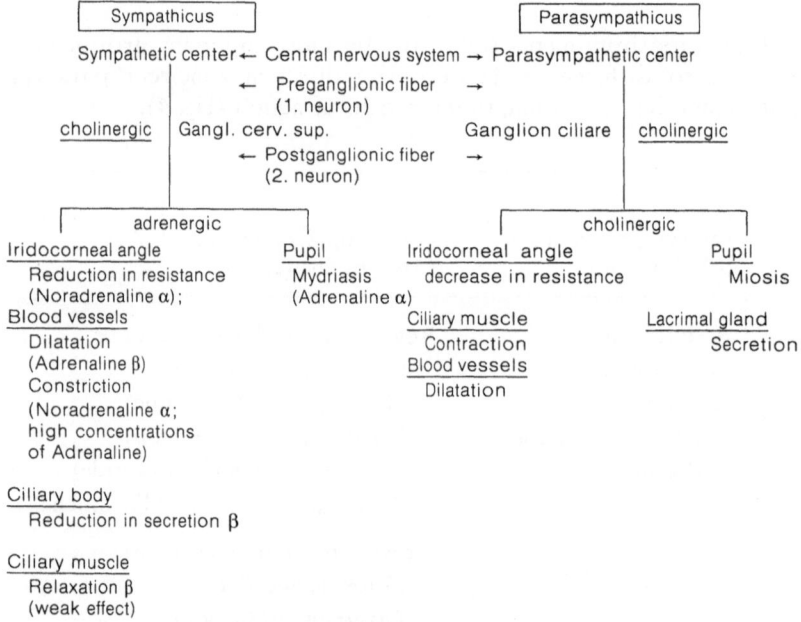

Fig. 5. Sympathicus and parasympathicus on the eye.
(Quoted from Heilmann)

The possible significance of this with regard to the rôle of blood supply to the optic nerve disk and its pressure tolerance is obvious. It follows that the range of application of sympathomimetics is narrowly restrictered and that a very accurate diagnosis is imperative when administering these.

Even the smaller dosage in the form of dipivalyl-epinefrine makes no difference to this point of view as, upon transformation of the prodrug in the eye, no lower concentration becomes active than with pure adrenaline preparations.

In the past decade drugs from the group of sympatholytics or antisympathotonics have been increasing in significance (Fig. 6).

Central	Reserpine
	—
	Clonidine
Ganglionic	Pendiomide
Postganglionic	6-Hydroxydopamine
	—
	α-Methyl-Dopa
	—
	Guanethidine, Reserpine
	—
	Dibenamine
	—
	Propranolol (β-blocker)

Fig. 6. Reduction in ocular pressure due to antisympathotonics

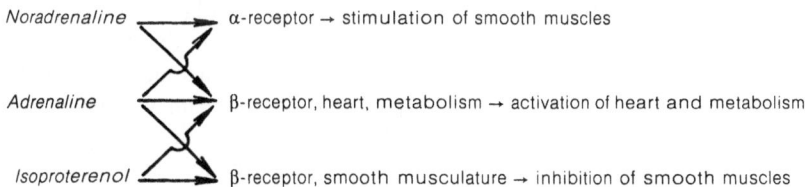

Fig. 7. Model for the effects of various catecholamines
(Kuschinski: Kurzes Lehrbuch der Pharmakologie und Toxikologie)

Two types of receptors are available for the transmission of sympathetic stimuli from the sympathetic nerve fiber end to the effector organ (Fig. 7). The smooth musculature is stimulated via alpha-receptors. Stimulation of the beta-1-receptors (e. g. in the cardiac musculature) and the beta-2-receptors in the intestinal musculature produces an impulse. Stimulation of the beta-2-receptors in the smooth muscle cells of the bronchi and vessels produces an inhibition of these muscle fibers.

The physiological transmitting substance noradrenaline mainly stimulates alpha-receptors and brings about a marked vasoconstriction. Adrenaline activates alpha- and beta-receptors and, according to the predominance of the alpha- or beta-receptor stimulus, provokes a vasoconstriction or vasodilatation. An influencing of the various receptors in the eye can produce a more or less pronounced reduction in pressure. Alpha-receptor blockers, such as dibenamine for example, used to be employed intravenously to reduce pressure in acute glaucoma. More recent studies show that selective stimulation of alpha-1-receptors causes an increase in ocular pressure accompanied by a mydriasis and a stimulation of alpha-2-receptors brings about distinct reduction in pressure dependent on dosage.

From the chemical point of view clonidine, a substance the mechanism and site of action of which has not been clarified, is related to the alpha-receptor blocking agents, for example tolazoline (Fig. 8).

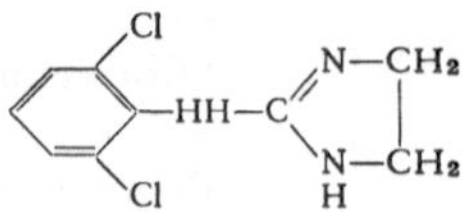

Fig. 8. Structural formula of clonidine

Clonidine produces a good reduction in ocular pressure and demonstrates excellent topical tolerance. A serious disadvantage is seen in that, contrary to most of the other antiglaucomatous agents, it is absorbed to a high degree by the blood stream via the nasal mucosa and digestive mucosa and can result in distinct systemic side effects. Especially in high concentrations dryness of the mouth, sedation, bradycardia and reduction in blood pressure can occur. Particularly this hypotensive side effect is in many cases not only undesirable but also possibly dangerous because of a potential deterioration of the circulatory situation at the optic nerve.

Yet another sympatholytic, guanethidine, has a direct effect on the terminal part of the sympathetic nerve fibers (Fig. 9). Due to a mobilisation of the granula and a thus increased release of noradrenaline (Fig. 10) there is at the beginning an increased outflow capacity because of the stimulation of alpha-receptors. This can be demonstrated tonographically. In the further course there occurs both an inhibition of the stimulus conduction and a depletion of noradrenaline in the sympathetic nerve ending. The subsequent reduction in ocular pressure ensues mainly via a reduction of aqueous secretion. Narrowing of the palpebral fissure and particularly rubor of the conjunctiva and the margins of the eye lids prevent a spreading of the substance. Further studies have demonstrated that adrenaline application following the administration of guanethidine produces a further decrease in ocular pressure and this led to the combination of these two substances at a smaller dosage than in single-dose treatment. A good reduction in pressure accompanied by a decrease in the side effects already mentioned resulted.

$$\bigcirc N-CH_2-CH_2-NH-C\begin{smallmatrix} NH_2 \\ \\ NH \end{smallmatrix}$$

Fig. 9. Structural formula of guanethidine (Ismeline)

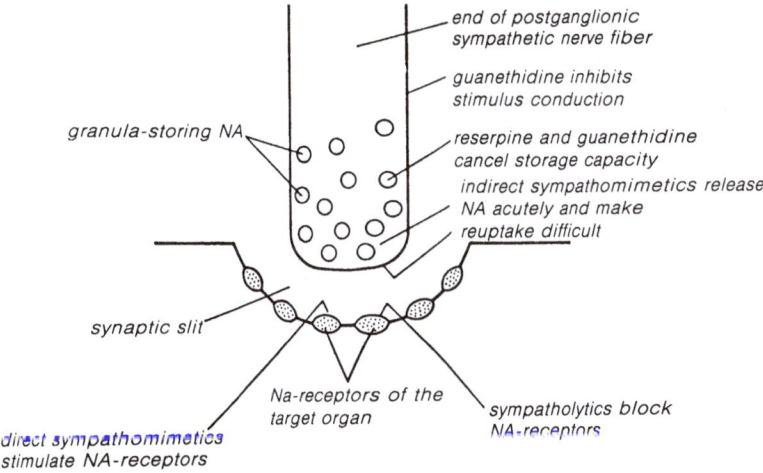

Fig. 10. Model for the action of sympathomimetics and antisympathotonics. (Kuschinski: Kurzes Lehrbuch der Pharmakologie und Toxikologie)

Particularly in the last few years beta-receptor blockers have been used widely in the treatment of chronic open-angle glaucoma. Human intraocular pressure is reduced, partly for a long duration, by local, oral and intravenous methods of application. The pharmacological differentiation of beta-blocking agents is concerned mainly with four characteristics (Fig. 11):

	First publication on usage as eye drops	Reducing intraocular pressure	Cardio-selectivity	Intrinsic sympathomimetic activity	Membrane activity
Propranolol (1%)	1968	+	−	−	+
Sotalol (2%)	1971	−	−	−	−
Practolol (10%)	1973	+	+	+	−
Oxprenolol (0.5%)	1975	+	−	+	+
Pindolol (1%)	1975	+	−	+	−
Atenolol (0.4%)	1976	+	+	−	−
Bupranolol (1%)	1976	+	−	−	+
Timolol (0.1—0.5%)	1976	+	−	−	−
Metoprolol	1977	+	+	−	+

Fig. 11. Beta-blocking agents tested for their suitability as antiglaucomatous agents

1. The beta-blocking strength; propranolol as reference substance is given as being equal to 1.
2. Membrane-stabilizing properties; many beta-blocking agents demonstrate membrane-stabilizing properties, i. e. their effect on eye is similar to that of a local anaesthetic.
3. Intrinsic sympathomimetic properties; beta-blocking agents with this property do not only cause a blocking but also exercise a slight stimulation on the receptors.
4. Selectivity; this denotes the presence or absence of a pharmacological affinity to the various beta-receptors.

At present it still cannot be said which structural characteristics and which spectrum of pharmacological properties predestines a beta-blocker for usage in glaucoma. The principal peculiarity of beta-blockers as opposed to miotics is that they are able to decrease ocular pressure in general, i. e. not only in glaucoma patients. Our own studies, carried out in cooperation with the first medical clinic of our university, plainly demonstrated such an effect upon the systemic administration of propranolol and metoprolol (Fig. 12). Furthermore it is worthy of note that beta-blocking agents do not show any effect on the width of pupil and accommodation.

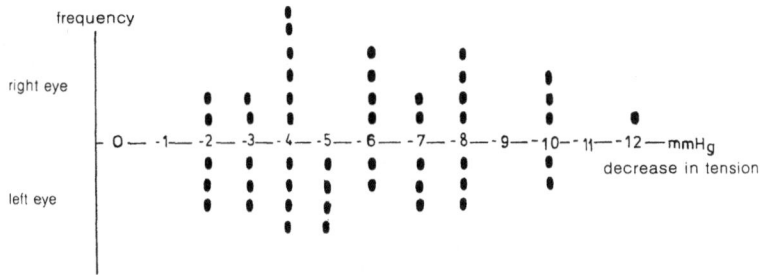

Fig. 12. Decrease in tension upon peroral treatment with Propranolol or Metoprolol on healthy eyes

Even if some studies give reason for the assumption that there is a slight influence on the capacity of aqueous outflow, the main mechanism still seems to be the diminishing of aqueous secretion. After a pronounced decrease in pressure at the beginning a distinct reduction of the pressure sinking effect is seen in the course of the first few days and weeks. Compared with an initial effect of almost 50%, in the most cases only a lasting reduction in pressure of 25% is shown and in the course of the further period of treatment this can decrease slightly but steadily. Damage to the corneal epithelium can be seen as local action on the eye due to the local anaesthetic effect mentioned. Also a decrease in lacrimal production and in rare instances allergisations were observed.

Particularly of late there have been loud warnings of a potential decrease in blood supply in the region of the optic nerve and of the danger of a so-called sanding of the trabecula after prolonged usage. This insolves a deterioration of the capacity of aqueous outflow due to the decrease in the flow of aqueous humour. Admittedly, such side effects have so far not been demonstrated but they cannot be ruled out.

With regard to systemic side effects a decrease in blood pressure and frequency of pulse, sensation of dizziness, depressions and cardiac asequence have been reported. Attacks of asthma can be triggered off by beta-2-inhibition in the bronchial tubes. Such observations, however, are relatively rare and with regard to topical application to the eye in the usual dosage they indicate a predisposition that would exclude the patient from this therapy. Despite the presence of these side effects beta-blockers represent a significant breakthrough in the treatment of chronic glaucomas. The subjective discomfort to the patient is decreased considerable or even completely compensated for by the absence of myosis and myopisation as well as by the prolonged duration of action upon application to the eye.

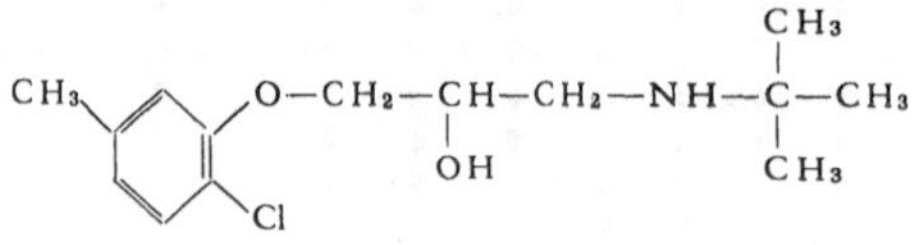

Bupranololum

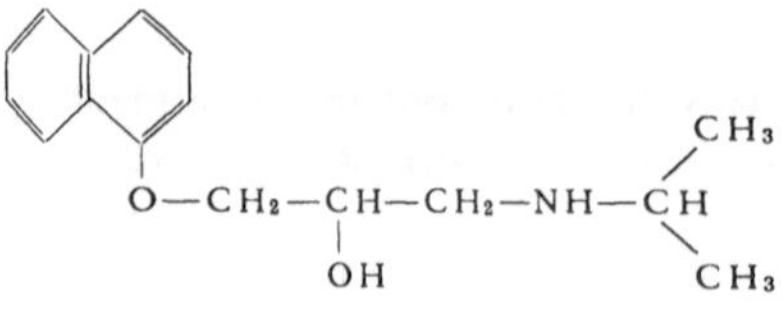

Propranololum

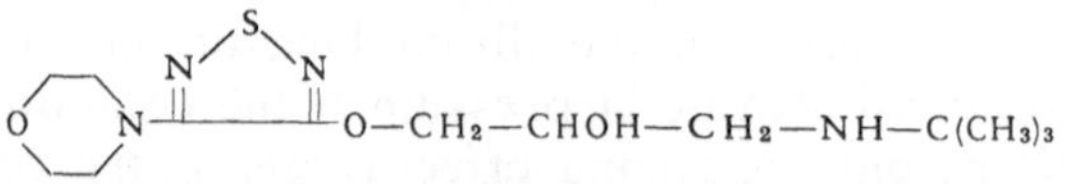

Timololum

Fig. 13. Structural formula of Bupranolol, Propranolol and Timolol

The reduction of ocular pressure with beta-blockers allows a more active participation in street traffic and makes it possible for the patient to continue his profession or to devote his time to his favourite hobby. Such activities are often considerably restricted due to the administration of miotics. Yet another advantage is that the patient is more willing to accept the regular instillation of these drops than of medicines with more serious subjective side effects.

The increase in the usage of beta-blockers within a comparatively short time due to the advantages described above has led to the search for newer, even more suitable substances form this group. Now that the experience of many years has been collected on the

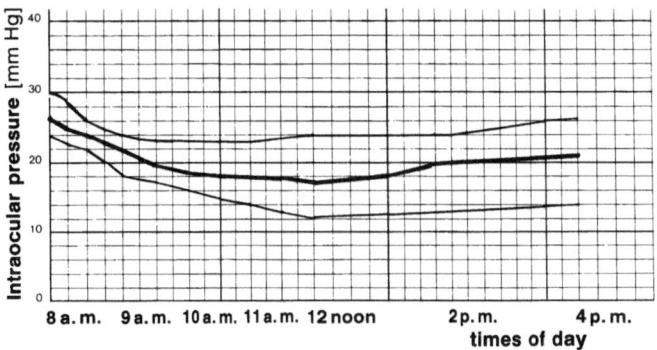

Fig. 14. Mean values and ranges of diffusion of pressure course upon single dosage of timolol

effect of propranolol, timolol and bupranol (Fig. 13). whereby timolol has generally proved to be the most suitable agent, clinical research has now proceeded to specialize in the search for new beta-sympatholytics. This search is directed at substances the side effects of which can be more calculated and the pressure reduction of which is more constant or higher at a lower dosage than is the case with those substances already being used. One part of the clinical studies — in our clinic for example — deals with the testing of new selective substances which block the beta-1-receptors only. There is reason to hope that this will involve less risk of an asthmatic attack occurring and also that a slighter decrease in blood supply will be achieved because of the selective blocking. Another part of the clinical studies is concerned with the so-called sterically pure beta-blockers, i. e. substances containing only the pharmacologically active part of the racemic mixture. In this case also one can hope for an increase in effect at a lower dosage as well as a decrease of side effects.

Such new substances to be tested are frequently compared with a substance of known and proven action instead of with a placebo. At present the preparation belonging to the group of beta-blockers which has been investigated most extensively is, without any doubt, timolol. This is why it is often used as a reference substance for comparison purposes. Metipranolol which is the main issue in most of the following papers was examined in our clinic and our study included the examination of its initial pressure reducing effect by means of one-drop curves. It was demonstrated with this small study that the reduction in pressure which a single dosage of metipranolol produces in a glaucomatous eye is more or less equivalent to the reduction in pressure obtained with timolol (Figs. 14 and 15).

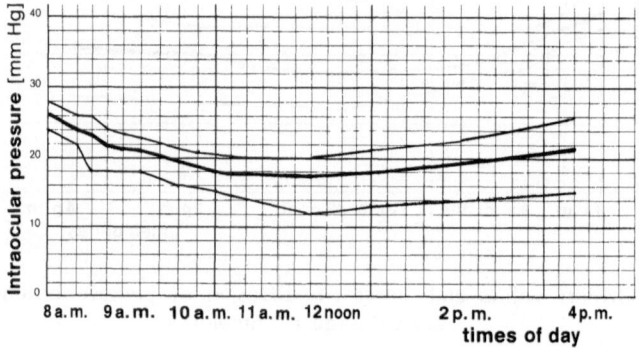

Fig. 15. Mean values and ranges of diffusion of pressure course upon single-dosage of metipranolol

Authors' address: Prof. Dr. H.-J. Merté, Augenklinik und -poliklinik rechts der Isar der Technischen Universität München, Ismaninger Strasse 22, D-8000 München 80, Federal Republic of Germany.

Pharmacological Spectrum of Metipranolol and Experience in Clinical Use

W. Bartsch, G. Sponer, and K. Strein

Department of Medical Research, Boehringer Mannheim GmbH, Mannheim, Federal Republic of Germany

With 6 Figures

Introduction

In the past few years β-receptor blockers have assumed a firm although not entirely undisputed position in the treatment of glaucomas. This indication came quite unexpectedly. When the ocular pressure of glaucoma patients who were receiving oral treatment with β-receptor blocking agents for other diseases, e. g. angina pectoris or hypertension, was measured a pressure reducing, i. e. therapeutic effect, was revealed [1, 2].

In 1899 Jonnesco published a paper entitled "Die Resektion des Halssympathikus in der Behandlung des Glaukoms" [3]. This early paper thus provided indications of an influence of the autonomic nervous system on intraocular pressure.

Although there does not exist any doubt nowadays that β-receptor blocking agents are able to reduce increased intraocular pressure, the mechanism of this therapeutic effect has — as far as we know — not been absolutely clarified, all the more so as both β-blocking agents and adrenergic stimulants (for example noradrenaline, dopamine, phenylephrine) can reduce elevated ocular pressure [4, 5]. Whereas it was originally assumed that the ocular pressure reducing property of β-blocking agents is related directly to a local anaesthetic or membrane-stabilizing property [6], we now know that this assumption is incorrect as substances without any local anaesthetic quality worth mentioning e. g. timolol (the following always refers to S-timolol) and metipranolol, reduce ocular pressure.

Furthermore it has been seen that too pronounced an anaesthetic quality is not only unnecessary but also limits tolerance. This is probably also the reason why β-blocking agents with an excessive anaesthetic quality are not used in the therapy of glaucoma.

Pharmacological Characterization of Metipranolol

β-receptor blockers, which are competitive antagonists may be characterized as follows:

1. Affinity to β-receptor, i. e. tendency to bind themselves to the receptor;
2. selectivity, i. e. the preferred antagonistic action on β_1 (cardiac) or β_2 (smooth-muscular, i. e. bronchial and vasal) receptors;
3. their intrinsic sympathomimetic action and
4. the membrane-stabilizing or surface-anaesthetic quality. The surface-anaesthetic property is undoubtedly of significance for the suitability of a β-blocker as a glaucoma treatment.

To be able to classify metipranolol in the spectrum of β-blocking agents you will find some physico-chemical characteristics along with the chemical structure in Table 1. In ophthalmological use the liposolubility (expressed as octanol/water quotient) should be of vital significance as an extremely hydrophilic or extremely lipophilic substance probably does not penetrate the various tissue layers so well as a β-blocker which is both hydrophilic and lipophilic. As can also be seen in Table 1, there are no relevant differences between the various β-blockers under discussion as far as their elimination kinetics are concerned [7—15]. It is questionable whether the differences in protein binding (between 10 and 93%) are of significance for topical application.

β-blocking Potency

It is possible to demonstrate the β-blockade and its potency in a wide variety of systems (isolated cells, isolated organs, anaesthetized or conscious animals and in humans).

The antagonism to the effect of the β-stimulant isoprenaline is by definition very suitable for characterization (see Bartsch et al., 1977 [16], for details on the method). The results illustrated in Fig. 1 show only relatively slight differences with regard to potency,

Table 1. *Chemical structure of the beta-blockers investigated and their protein binding, liposolubility and duration of action*

SUBSTANCE	Ar - O - CH$_2$- CHOH - CH$_2$ - NH - R		Mol-weight (Base)	Protein binding %	Distribution ratio octanol/water pH 7	Elimination half life t/2 (h)
	Ar	R				
Alprenolol	(CH$_2$-CH=CH$_2$)	CH (CH$_3$)$_2$	249.3	85 (7)	3,27 (10)	2 - 5 (8)
Bupranolol *	Cl—CH$_3$	C (CH$_3$)$_3$	271.8	—	3,75 (10)	2 - 4 (8,11)
Metipranolol *	H$_3$C—CH$_3$, CH$_3$ O-CO-CH$_3$		309.4	70	0,68	3 - 4 (12)
Pindolol	(N H)	CH (CH$_3$)$_2$	248.3	57 (15)	0,20 (10)	3 - 5 (9)
Propranolol			259.3	93 (7)	5,40 (7)	2 - 5 (9)
S - Timolol *	O N—N N S	C (CH$_3$)$_3$	316.4	10 (15)	0,51 (13)	2 - 5 (9)

* = available as eye drops; ( ) = literature reference

i. e. the β-blocking equipotent doses. The inhibition of a rate increase under isoprenaline (1 mcg/kg i. v. increased heart rate from about 220 to about 340 beats/minute) was measured on the conscious rabbit. The results of this test are given in Table 2.

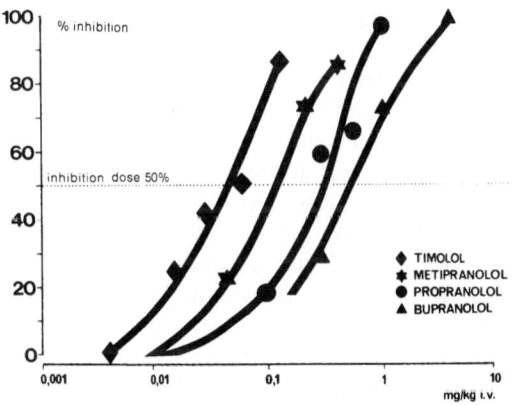

Fig. 1. Inhibition of increase in heart rate following isoprenaline (1 mcg/kg i. v.) in the conscious rabbit. (The values of the equipotent beta-blocking doses are to be found in Table 2)

In the same experimental model, using metipranolol as an example, Fig. 2 illustrates the competitive antagonism, to adrenergic stimulation, which is valid for all β-blocking agents in the same manner.

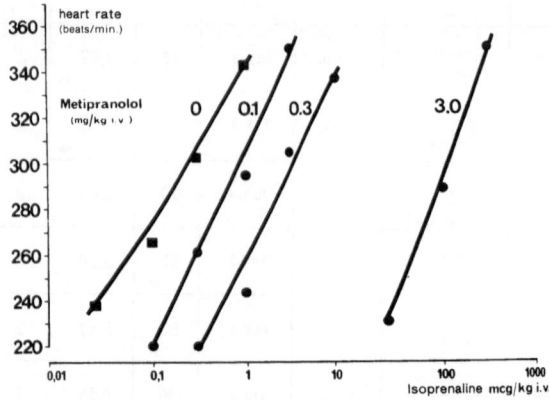

Fig. 2. Shift to the right of dose response curves of isoprenaline produced by metipranolol in conscious rabbit; competitive antagonism

This means that the effect of the β-blocking agent can be overcome by an increase of the agonist dose (in this example that of isoprenaline, by noradrenaline in the body).

Intrinsic Sympathomimetic Activity (ISA)

Rats which have been especially sensitized to stimulating influences by means of catecholamine depletion (5 mg/kg s. c. reserpine dose 24 hours before) are suitable for detecting ISA (= intrinsic sympathomimetric activity). In this way it is possible to detect sympathomimetic — i. e. rate increasing — effects of β-blockers even when such effects are present at a very low degree. These studies, which are carried out according to the Barrett/Carter-method [17] provided, if the equipotent β-blocking doses are taken into consideration, information on the extent of the sympathomimetic action. The basal rate of these catecholamine-depleted rats is about 270 beats/minute. The values shown in Fig. 3 refer to the increase of heart rate compared with the basal rate. Apart from pindolol, none of the β-blockers examined showed any noteworthy intrinsic sympathomimetic activity.

The clinical relevance of this activity in internal medicine is disputed [18, 19] and it is unknown up to now in ophthalmology.

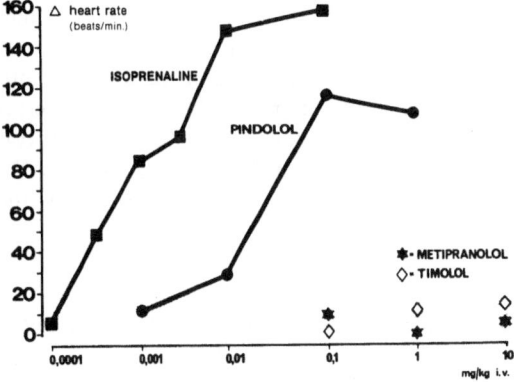

Fig. 3. Intrinsic sympathomimetic activity, increase of heart rate of conscious rates pretreated with reserpine (5 mg/kg s. c. 24 hours before) following the administration of various beta-blockers compared with the beta-stimulant isoprenaline

Surface Anaesthetic Activity
(also Membrane-stabilizing Activity — MSA)

To determine this activity the rabbit cornea was stimulated mechanically (impulse rate 50/min, pressure 200 mg) and the concentration at which 50 stimuli were required to produce a blink was determined [20].

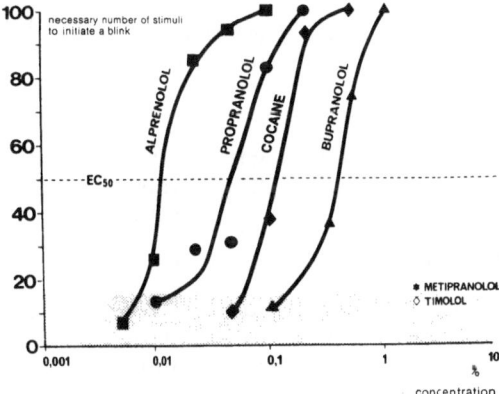

Fig. 4. Dose response curves for surface anaesthesia of the rabbit cornea for various beta-blockers and cocaine as well as the absence of this property for timolol and metipranolol

W. Bartsch, G. Sponer, and K. Strein:

Whereas alprenolol and propranolol have an anaesthetic effect even at lower concentrations than cocaine, timolol and metipranolol are different in that no relevant anaesthesia is detectable up to a concentration of 2% (Fig. 4). This does not mean that the action is not present at all, but only that a grading of action in relation to concentration cannot be determined. Higher concentrations produce problems of solubility, particularly as only certain pharmaceutical preparations can be considered for administration to the eye, as will be dealt with later in the contribution by Wawretschek. For example, osmolarity and the pH must be kept within relatively narrow limits.

Table 2. *Quantitative comparison of the qualities of action of various β-blockers*

| Substance | β-Blockade | | ISA % | MSA EC_{50} % | $\frac{EC_{50}}{ID_{50}}$ | Relation Bupranolol = 1 |
	ID_{50} (mg/kg i. v.)	RP Propranolol = 1				
Alprenolol	0.437	0.44	<10	0.012	0.027	0.03
Bupranolol	0.448	0.43	<10	0.36	0.804	1.00
Metipranolol	0.109	1.77	<10	>3.0	>27.5	>34.2
Pindolol	0.077	2.51	~60	0.12	1.558	1.94
Propranolol	0.193	1.00	~10	0.055	0.285	0.35
Timolol	0.041	4.71	<10	>2.0	>48.7	>60.5

ID_{50} = Measure of the β-blockade, dose for the inhibition of isoprenaline tachycardia (1 mcg/kg i. v.) by 50%.

RP = Potency relative to propranolol.

ISA = Intrinsic rate increasing activity as a percent of a maximum isoprenaline effect in rats pretreated with reserpine (5 mg/kg s. c., 24 hours before) at ID_{50}.

MSA = Membrane stabilizing activity.

EC_{50} = Measure of the surface anaesthesia, effective concentration in percent at which the stimulation of the cornea responds with blinking only after 50 impulses.

$EC_{50} : ID_{50}$ = Anaesthetic potency in relation to β-blocking potency; relation bupranolol = 1 — high figures indicate a lower surface anaesthetic action than bupranolol.

Cardioselectivity

The pharmacological characteristics can be obtained clearly in isolated cells or isolated organs from the ratio of the cardiac (β_1) to the bronchial or vasal (β_2) β-blockade. In the following a detailed presentation of these results will be dispensed with, as all the β-blockers examined are classifiable as non-selective. Occasionally it has been claimed that the β-blocking agent metipranolol is cardioselective [21, 22], but better founded results of experiments (Lundgren et al. [23] as well as unpublished results of our own) contradict this assessment and show that metipranolol has a balanced ratio of the β-blockade $(\beta_1 : \beta_2)$.

A summary of the pharmacological characteristics is given in Table 2, whereby the β-blocking active dose is also shown in comparison with propranolol as this β-blocker is the best known. The surface anaesthetic concentration was determined as an absolute value (column MSA EC_{50} in percent) and related to the β-blocking active dose.

A comparison was also made with bupranolol $(= 1)$ as this β-blocker is marketed as a treatment for glaucoma but still possesses an anaesthetic property which is clearly measurable.

Reduction of Ocular Pressure

There can be little doubt that findings concerning the reduction of intraocular pressure (IOP) by β-blocking agents are of interest to ophthalmologists. In contrast to experimental findings with various β-blocking agents on models with increased IOP [24—27], Cepelik and Dienstbier jr. [28] have recently published results with metipranolol used topically in rabbits with normal IOP.

It was found that ocular pressure was reduced, but that the reduction (see Fig. 5) was only significant with the 2% metipranolol solution ($p < 0.05$). Also in the case of timolol [29] a reduction in pressure in animals with normal IOP was obtained only at relatively high concentrations (2 and 4%). Although the reduction in ocular pressure in the rabbit was only moderate and occurred only at a relatively high concentration, there is nevertheless a direct relation to the therapeutically desired action.

When considering these results it must be borne in mind that the model described above begins with normal pressure and, therefore, very distinctive effects are not to be expected [30].

This provides a parallel to arterial blood pressure which, provided it is in the normal range, is scarcely reduced by β-blocking agents. This applies to studies in humans and even more distinctly to those in animals with systemic administration.

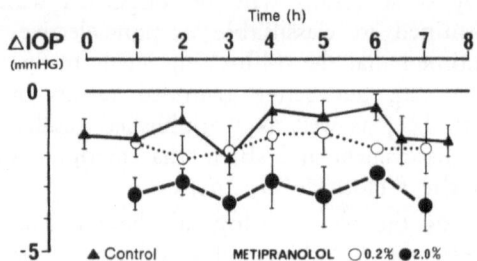

Fig. 5. Reduction of normal ocular pressure in albino rabbits after 0.2 % and 2.0 % metipranolol eye drops (n = 8). (Cepelik and Dienstbier [28])

Experience in Clinical Therapy and Tolerance

The β-blocking agent metipranolol is available on the German market as Disorat in tablets of 10 and 20 mg. The indications are coronary heart diseases (angina pectoris), cardiac autonomic dysregulation, cardiac arrhythmia, hyperkinetic heart syndrome, and arterial hypertension.

Furthermore, a combination product containing metipranolol 20 mg with the diuretic butizide 2.5 mg is marketed in Germany as Torrat® and since 1982 as Tri-Torrat® which contains metipranolol 20 mg + butizide 2.5 mg + dihydralazine 25 mg.

Sufficient publications [31—41] have been produced on the therapeutic effects of metipranolol and its combinations in various indications, so that there is no need to go into that here.

As far as the ophthalmologist is concerned, a point of contact with the internal specialist is, no doubt, the diagnosis "Fundus hypertonicus" (see Fig. 6), i. e. the changes in the ocular fundus which appear in the course of arterial hypertension.

As very extensive and, in part, relatively new clinical results are available with metipranolol in this respect, I should now like to report on the rate of success in the treatment of hypertension using the β-blocking agent metipranolol alone or with its combinations [42, 43].

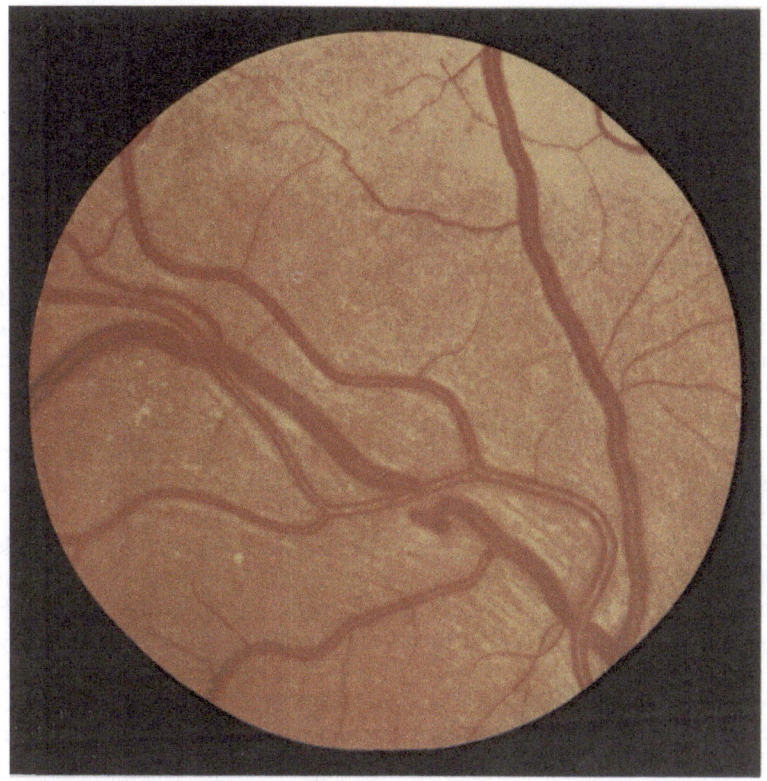

Fig. 6. Fundus hyperthonicus
From: Der Augenhintergrund, p. 116, Fig. 100. Stuttgart — New York:
Schattauer. 1980. (Reproduced with permission of the publishers)

Frequency of success in patients in whom a reduction of blood
pressure to diastolic values of less than 95 mmHg was achieved
(1—3 tablets daily):

Metipranolol 20 mg $= 64\%$
(= Disorat®)

Metipranolol 20 mg + butizide 2.5 mg $= 84\%$
(= Torrat®)

Metipranolol 20 mg + butizide 2.5 mg + dihydralazine 25 mg $= 92\%$
(= Tri-Torrat®)

The question of the occurrence of side effects is of particular
interest, even if conclusions with regard to the risks of topical

application can only be drawn to a very limited extent from experience made with oral administration.

Tolerance and Potential of Side Effects

The type and frequency of side effects do not differ from those of other β-blocking substances [41, 42].

According to the information reaching the manufacturer the main side effects are: gastrointestinal intolerance, bradycardia, feeling of dizziness, orthostatic dysregulations and occasionally skin reactions and headache. Some of the side effects which have been reported (orthostatic dysregulation, status asthmaticus, bradycardia) can easily be related to the β-blocking action, others, such as potency disorders, sedation and increase in uric acid, are, in part, difficult to associate with therapy and the underlying disease or the therapeutic principle of β-blockade.

In the following some comments are made with regard to the risk of side effects on topical administration of metipranolol. 1 ml of the 0.6% solution has about 30 drops. If 1 drop is instilled into each eye the total amount of metipranolol is about 400 mcg. Assuming the least probable case that the total β-blocker amount is absorbed either in the eye or via the ductus nasolacrimalis, one may ask what effects or side effects are to be expected with an i. v. administration of this quantity of the substance and upon the administration of higher doses. According to an in-house report by the manufacturers [44] dealing with the examination for bioavailability (result 50 %) doses of 6—25 mg metipranolol per test person, slowly infused, ($n = 27$), were, without exception, tolerated well. However, it must be granted that this was a clinical pharmacological study with healthy persons, i. e. actual patients were excluded from the test.

Although one might actually presume that upon the administration of β-blockers as eye drops effects other than on the eye are not to be expected because of the low quantity of the drug, experience with timolol [45, 46, 47) has shown that systemic side effects can occur on topical application. Therefore, and unfortunately this must be emphasized, when prescribing β-blockers in the form of eye drops, one has no choice but either to exclude patients with contra-indications (asthma, broncho-obstructive diseases, AV-block as well as latent and manifest heart failure) from therapy or at least to proceed with the utmost caution.

In many cases contact with the internal specialist might prove useful.

Now that I have tried to characterize the spectrum of action of metipranolol and have passed some comments with regard to the occurrence of side effects I should, in conclusion, like to quote from Jonnesco's paper which I mentioned at the beginning [3]. He wrote 83 years ago:

"that only then, when the nervous mechanism of the intraocular secretions or, to speak without hypothesis, the action of the nervous system on the intraocular pressure is known, will the pathogenesis of glaucoma be clear, iridectomy be explained and a new treatment of glaucoma — perhaps on a scientific basis — be founded."

One might well assume that the author had an idea, however vague, of these substances in the sense of the sympatholysis. Did he, when writing that, have drugs like timolol and metipranolol in mind?

Acknowledgement

We should like to thank Rhein-Pharma, Merck, Sharp and Dohme, and Sandoz for supplying us with the test substances propranolol, S-timolol and pindolol. In particular we wish to thank the following members of staff: E. Dietz, G. Gebhardt, B. Gessel, J. Janich, M. Kohler, and A. Litters.

References

1. Phillips, C. I., Howitt, G., Rowlands, D. L.: Propranolol as ocular hypotensive agent. Br. J. Ophthalmol. 51, 222—226 (1967).

2. Wettrell, K., Pandolfi, M.: Propranolol vs. acetazolamide. A long-term double masked study of the effect on intraocular pressure and blood-pressure. Arch. Ophthalmol. 97, 280—283 (1979).

3. Jonnesco, T.: Die Resection des Halssympathicus in der Behandlung des Glaukoma. Wien. klin. Wschr. 12, 483—486 (1899).

4. Potter, D. E.: Adrenergic pharmacology of aqueous humor dynamics. Pharmacol. Rev. 33, 133—153 (1981).

5. Kahan, A.: Miscellaneous effects: Effects of adrenergic activators and inhibitors on the eye. In: Handbook of Experimental Pharmacology, Vol. 54: Adrenergic Activators and Inhibitors, Part II (Szekeres, L., ed.), pp. 319—344. Berlin—Heidelberg—New York: Springer. 1981.

6. Bucci, M. G., Missiroli, A., Giraldi, J., Virno, M.: Local administration of propranolol in the treatment of glaucoma. Boll. Oculist. 47, 51—60 (1968).

7. Johnsson, G., Regardh, C.-G.: Clinical pharmacokinetics of β-adreno-receptor blocking drugs. Clin. Pharmacokin. 1, 233—263 (1976).

8. Gugler, R.: Pharmakokinetische Unterschiede zwischen β-Rezeptoren-blockern. In: Beta-Rezeptorenblocker (Bolte, H.-D., Schrey, A., eds.), pp. 19—22. Berlin — Heidelberg — New York. 1981.

9. Shanks, R. G.: Pharmacokinetics of beta-receptor-blocking drugs. In: Differenzierte Therapie mit Beta-Rezeptorenblockern (Symposium, Lissabon, 25. und 26. September 1980) (Palm, D., Stein, U., eds.), pp. 63—68. Heidelberg: Rausch. 1982.

10. Hellenbrecht, D., Gortner, L.: Correlations between hydrophobicity and non-specific pharmacological effects of β-adrenoceptor blocking agents. Pol. J. Pharmacol. Pharm. 28, 625—630 (1976).

11. Seyfried, Chr.: Zur Pharmakokinetik und relativen Bioverfügbarkeit von Metipranolol bei Leberzirrhotikern unterschiedlichen Schwere-grades. Dissertation, Berlin, 1981.

12. Seyfried, Chr., Ledermann, H., Rennekamp, H., L'Age, M., Abshagen, U.: Pharmakokinetik des β-Rezeptorenblockers Metipranolol bei Patienten mit Leberzirrhose. Dtsch. med. Wschr. 107, 21—26 (1982).

13. Woods, P. B., Robinson, M. L.: An investigation of the comparative liposolubilities of β-adrenoceptor blocking agents. J. Pharm. Pharmacol. 33, 172—173 (1981).

14. Knauf, H., Schäfer-Korting, M., Mutschler, E.: Pharmakokinetik und biologische Wirkdauer von β-Rezeptorenblockern bei Niereninsuffizienz. Internist 22, 616—621 (1981).

15. Dunn, F. G., Frohlich, E. D.: Pharmacokinetics, mechanisms of action, indications, and adverse effects to timolol maleate, a non-selective beta-adrenoceptor blocking agent. Pharmacotherapy 1, 188—200 (1981).

16. Bartsch, W., Sponer, G., Dietmann, K.: Experiments in animals on the pharmacological effects of metipranolol in comparison with propranolol and pindolol. Arzneim.-Forsch./Drug Res. 27, 2319—2322 (1977).

17. Barrett, A. M., Carter, J.: Comparative chronotropic activity of β-adrenoceptive antagonists. Brit. J. Pharmacol. 40, 373—381 (1970).

18. Cocco, G., Burkart, F., Chu, D., Follath, F.: Intrinsic sympathomimetic activity of β-adrenoceptor blocking agents. Europ. J. clin. Pharmacol. 13, 1—4 (1978).

19. Noack, E.: Intrinsische sympathomimetische Aktivität bei Beta-Rezeptorenblockern. Münch. med. Wschr. 124, 377—380 (1982).

20. Bartsch, W., Knopf, K.-W.: Eine modifizierte Methode zur Prüfung der Oberflächenanästhesie an der Kaninchen-Cornea. Arzneim.-Forsch./Drug Res. 20, 1140—1143 (1970).

21. Rascher, W., Mann, J. F. E., Schömig, A., Dietz, R., Lüth, J. B.: Effects of β-adrenergic blocking agents on peripheral vascular resistance. Klin. Wschr. 56 (Suppl. I), 87—90 (1978).

22. Kather, H., Simon, B.: β-blocking agents and human fat cell adenylate cyclase. Res. Comm. Chem. Path. Pharmacol. 18, 11—22 (1977).

23. Lundgren, B., Carlsson, E., Ablad, B.: Pharmakologischer Nachweis der β_1-Selektivität von β-Rezeptorenblockern. Med. Welt 29, 1531 (1978).

24. Bonomi, L., Perfetti, S., Noya, E., Bellucci, R., Massa, F.: Comparison of the effects of nine beta-adrenergic blocking agents on intraocular pressure in rabbits. Graefes Arch. Klin. Exp. Ophthalmol. 10, 1—8 (1979).

25. Liu, H. K., Chiou, G. C. Y., Garg, L. C.: Ocular hypotensive effects of timolol in cat eyes. Arch. Ophthalmol. 98, 1467—1469 (1980).

26. McDonald, T. O., Hodges, J. W., Borgmann, A. R., Leaders, F. E.: The water-loading test in rabbits. Arch. Ophthalmol. 82, 381—384 (1969).

27. Vareilles, P., Silverstone, D., Plazonnet, B., Le Douarec, J.-C., Sears, M. L., Stone, C. A.: Comparison of the effects of timolol and other adrenergic agents on intraocular pressure in the rabbit. Invest. Ophthalmol. Visual Sci. 16/11, 987—996 (1977).

28. Cepelik, J., Dienstbier, E., jr.: Effects of adrenergic stimulating and blocking agents on intraocular pressure in the rabbit. Glaucoma 4, 216—224 (1982).

29. Colasanti, B. K., Trotter, R. R.: Effects of selective beta$_1$- and beta$_2$-adrenoreceptor agonists and antagonists on intraocular pressure in the cat. Invest. Ophthalmol. Visual Sci. 20, 69—76 (1981).

30. Nielsen, N. V.: Timolol and Metoprolol. Okulärer hypotensiver Effekt, lokale und systemische Begleiteffekte. Z. prakt. Augenheilkd. 2, 71—77 (1981).

31. Blömeke, H.: Untersuchung der antihypertensiven Wirksamkeit der einzelnen Komponenten von Torrat. Therapiewoche 30, 5523—5527 (1980).

32. Faupel, R. P., Gotzen, R.: Antihypertensive Langzeitbehandlung mit Torrat®. Med. Klin. 74, 929—934 (1979).

33. Greding, H., Doering, W., Isbary, J., Finger-Ishii, K., König, E.: Hämodynamische Veränderungen nach kombinierter oraler Gabe von Metipranolol und Isosorbiddinitrat bei Patienten mit koronarer Herzerkrankung. Herz/Kreisl. 12, 490—498 (1980).

34. Hayduk, K., Christ, H., Krauss, J., Halank, Chr., Kühn, A.: Intraindividueller Wirkungsvergleich der Einzelkomponenten mit einer fixen Betablocker-Thiazid-Kombination in der Behandlung der Hypertonie. Therapiewoche 29, 7528—7532 (1979).

35. Hopf, R., Tourbier, H., Kaltenbach, M.: Wirksamkeit des β-Sympathikolytikums Methypranol auf Belastungsherzfrequenz und ischämische ST-Senkung im Vergleich mit Placebo und Propranolol. Herz/Kreisl. 9, 560—565 (1977).

36. Franz, I.-W., Lohmann, F. W.: Der Einfluß einer Saluretikum-β-Rezeptorenblocker-Kombination auf überhöhte Belastungsblutdrücke. Med. Klin. 74, 396—400 (1979).

37. Janka, H. U., Standl, R., Vollmar, J., Bauer, G., Mehnert, H.: Der Einfluß einer antihypertensiven Kombinationstherapie auf den Stoffwechsel von Diabetikern. Ther. d. Gegenw. *119,* 74—89 (1980).

38. Kolloch, R., Overlack, A., Stumpe, K. O.: Antihypertensive Therapie mit einer fixen Beta-Rezeptorenblocker-Diuretikum-Kombination. Ther. d. Gegenw. *118,* 1517—1528 (1979).

39. Manteuffel, G. E. von, Ebel, H., Zehner, J.: Kombinationstherapie der arteriellen Hypertonie. Med. Klin. *75,* 297—302 (1980).

40. Mattern, Hj.: Dauerbehandlung der Hypertonie mit Torrat®: Vergleich der Wirksamkeit und Verträglichkeit bei fraktionierter und einmaliger Tagesgabe, Therapiewoche *28,* 2020—2027 (1978).

41. Schweers, A., Glocke, M., Smolarz, A., Timmler, R.: Langzeitbeobachtung der Hypertoniebehandlung mit Torrat®. Therapiewoche *28,* 8865—8872 (1978).

42. Smolarz, A.: 12 Monate Langzeitverträglichkeit eines β-Blockers. In: Klinische Pharmakologie und experimentelle Medizin, Vol. VI (Vogt, W., Boch, H. E., eds.), pp. 80—100. Aulendorff: Editio Cantor. 1980.

43. Smolarz, A.: Klinische Prüfung der Kombination Metipranolol, Butizid und Dihydralazin. In preparation (1983).

44. Abshagen, U., Betzien, G.: Zur Pharmakokinetik von Metipranolol bei gesunden freiwilligen Versuchspersonen. Int. Prüfbericht Boehringer Mannheim GmbH, 26. August 1980.

45. Williams, T., Ginther, W. H.: Hazard of ophthalmic timolol. New Engl. J. Med. *306,* 1485—1486 (1982).

46. Vonwil, A., Landolt, M., Flammer, J., Bachofen, H.: Bronchokonstriktive Nebenwirkungen von Timolol-Augentropfen bei Patienten mit obstruktiven Augenerkrankungen. Schweiz. Med. Wschr. *11,* 665—669 (1981).

47. Van Buskirk, E. M.: Adverse reactions from timolol administration. Ophthalmol. *87,* 447—450 (1980).

Authors' address: Dr. W. Bartsch, Messrs. Boehringer Mannheim GmbH, Sandhofer Strasse 116, D-6800 Mannheim 31, Federal Republic of Germany.

Suitability of Metipranolol for Glaucoma Therapy from the Pharmacological Viewpoint

Pharmacological Properties of Metipranolol in Glaucoma Therapy

E. A. Noack

Institute of Pharmacology,
University of Düsseldorf, Federal Republic of Germany

With 5 Figures

In the title of this report I mention the suitability of Metipranolol. What I mean is the usefulness of this beta-receptor blocking agent in topical administration to the eye, judged on the basis of its pharmacological properties but not with reference to efficacy from the clinical viewpoint. Beta-receptor blocking agents have now been used successfully for 15 years in glaucoma and to my understanding there cannot be any doubt about the basis efficacy of all beta-blocking agents which are on the market for this form of therapy.

The discovery of the antiglaucomatous action of beta-receptor blockers goes back to accidental observation by Phillips et al. [1] in 1967. When using propranolol systematically, this working group noticed that shortly after therapy had begun the glaucoma patients in their group of patients felt a subjective relief which turned out to be the result of a reduction in intraocular pressure.

Later Wetrell and Pandolfi [2] reported about comparative therapeutic success upon the oral administration of propranolol, whereby the test was already carried out as a double-blind cross-over study. McDonald et al. [3] and Elliot et al. [4] made similar reports upon using atenolol orally.

The hypotensive effects, however, proved to be even more pronounced when the beta-receptor blockers were applied topically to the eye.

In 1968 Bucci *et al.* [5] were the first to report on therapeutic success with the topical application of propranolol. One of the advantages of topical application is that only very small quantities of the active substance are necessary for an effective reduction in pressure. Provided these are absorbed by the general circulation, no systemic effects or only very slight systemic effects are to be expected. Only 0.17 mg of the active ingredient is contained in 1 drop of metipranolol eye drops 0.3 %.

It is typical that the reduction in intraocular pressure occurs even after a single application [6], whereby there are distinct sub-stance-specific differences in the intensity and duration of action [6—9] of the individual beta-receptor blocking agents. This is due to the fact that, apart from their specific beta-adrenolytical component of action, beta-receptor blocking agents possess more or less pronounced side effects which may restrict topical application and, also with regard to therapeutic aspects, this makes a comparison interesting.

In this respect I am thinking of properties such as the local an-aesthetic and membrane-stabilizing activity, cardioselectivity, a po-tential intrinsic sympathomimetic activity (ISA) and the extent of lipophilicity.

Apart from metipranolol, bupranolol under the brand name Ophtorenin® and timolol under the name Chibro-Timoptol® have so far been launched on the German pharmaceutical market. Fig. 1 shows the structural formulae of these beta-receptor blocking agents. I shall concentrate my report on the comparison of the pharma-cological properties of these substances in particular.

A major problem in the assessment of therapy with beta-receptor blocking agents is that there is still no clarity about the real mecha-nism of action underlying the reduction in intraocular pressure. This is also obvious from the very conflicting reports which were made in this respect at the Symposium der Deutschen Ophthalmolo-gischen Gesellschaft in April of last year [11]. In my opinion, the reason is that two very different qualities of action of beta-receptor blockers, namely their specific beta-adrenolytic action on the one hand and their unspecific local-anaesthetic activity on the other hand, may basically be made responsible for the reduction in pressure as experimental findings exist for both mechanisms, supporting their pharmacodynamic significance.

From the functional point of view there is a much clearer picture for the mechanism of the reduction in intraocular pressure. Many studies prove consistently and beyond doubt that beta-receptor blocking agents reduce aqueous production as a result of an inhibition of the active transport mechanisms in the ciliary epithelium. There are findings about a simultaneous influence on the facility of aqueous outflow but these are very controversial and do not allow any final judgement.

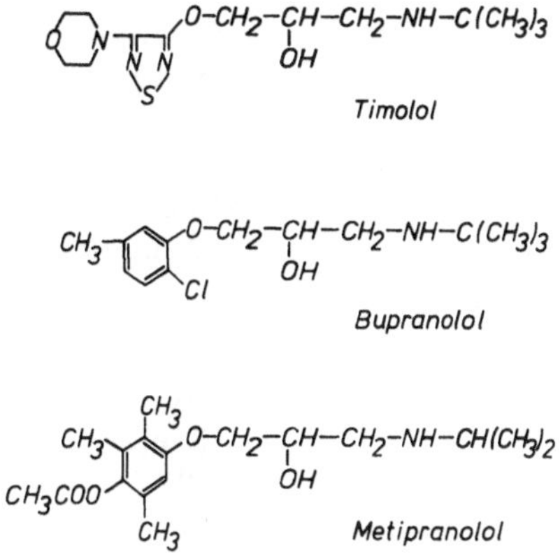

Fig. 1. Structural formulae of beta-receptor blockers which have already been introduced to the market in the Federal Republic of Germany for glaucoma therapy

Thus there are reports on facility [12—15], no influence [16, 17] and also an inhibition [18]. The fact that D-isomers of beta-receptor blocking agents, which demonstrate 50—100 times less binding affinity to the beta-receptor, do not trigger off any hypotensive effect whatsoever, speaks in favour of a specific receptor-mediated onset of action.

On the basis of comparative in-vitro studies by Kern [12] with muscle stripe preparations from the M. sphincter pupillae and M. ciliaris and from papers by other authors it is known that α- and β-adrenergic receptors are present both in the region of the M. ciliaris and the ciliary gland. By means of differential influencing of the ultrafiltration and aqueous secretion these can influence the level of intraocular pressure in an opposite way, whereby it is noticeable that the α-adrenergic receptors surpass the β-adrenergic both functionally and in terms of number. Stimulation of the α-adrenergic receptors induces — on the basis of experimental findings in the ciliary gland — a decrease in aqueous production as does the blockade of beta-receptors. This is a theoretical explanation why not only sympathomimetics of the type of adrenaline produce a reduction in intraocular pressure via a preferred stimulation of α-receptors but also sympatholytics of the type of metipranolol produce a reduction in like manner via a blockade of the β-adrenergic receptors, although this would seem paradoxical at a first glance. At the same time this explains the additive increase in effect upon cumulative use [8, 19]. Findings recently published by Innemee *et al.* [20] likewise suggest an opposing regulation of aqueous production in the range of the ciliary epithelium due to α- and β-receptors.

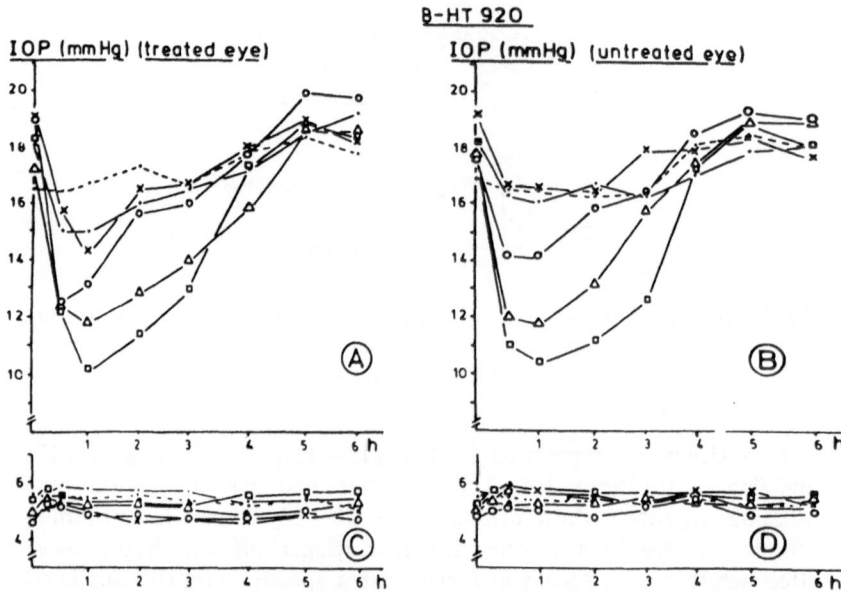

Fig. 2. Influence of B-HT 920 on intraocular pressure (*A* and *B*) and width of pupils (*C* and *D*) upon topical application of 50 μl to the right eye of the conscious rabbit. (•---•) physiological saline; (•—•) 0.01 %; (x—x) 0.03 % (○—○) 0.1 %; (△—△) 0.3 %; (□—□) 1 % B-HT 920. The symbols represent the mean values $\bar{x}$ ($n = 6$). Medium error of mean value $s_{\bar{x}} < 10$ %. (From Innemee et al., 1981 [20])

By means of comparison these authors studied the intraocular changes in pressure in the conscious rabbit upon topical application of selective α_1 and α_2 agonists and antagonists. They were able to differentiate the α-effect further in that they found that the selective stimulation of the α_1-receptor sub-type produced an increase in intraocular pressure with (−)-phenylephrine whereas the α_2-subtypes (DHT 920 and 933) led to a distinctive hypotensive reaction which could be completely offset again by the selective α_2-receptor antagonist yohimbine. Figs. 2 and 3 illustrate these findings.

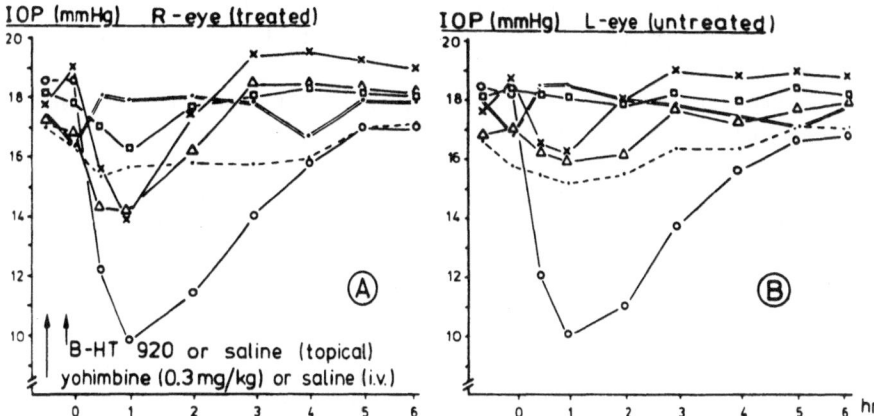

Fig. 3. Temporal course of intraocular reduction in pressure upon topical application of B-HT 920 in treated (A) and untreated (B) eye of conscious rabbit upon intravenous pretreatment with 0.3 mg of yohimbine/kg body weight. (• - - - •) physiological saline; (• = •) yohimbine (0.3 mg/kg i. v.) alone; (□—□) B-HT 920 (0.03 %) after yohimbine; (x—x) B-HT 920 (0.3 %) after yohimbine; (○—○) B-HT 920 (1 %) after yohimbine. Mean values of 6 animals. Medium error of mean value < 10 %. From Innemee et al., 1981, [20])

In this connection it is interesting that Neufeld and Page [21] and also Mittag and Tormay [22] demonstrated a prevalence of α_2-receptors in the region of the ciliary gland and iris by means of ligand binding studies. In addition Dafnar et al. [23] and Bromberg et al. [24] demonstrate a large β-receptor density in the region of the ciliary epithelium, which could be classified as mainly representing the β_2-subtype (Nathanson [25]). Despite the complexity of the underlying mechanism these findings indicate that a reduction in intraocular pressure can be mediated specifically by adrenergic receptors, be it by stimulation of α_2-receptors or by inhibition of β-receptors [26]. For the purposes of our review it is of little relevance whether this pharmacological influence on the adrenergic receptors is ultimately caused by a direct functional impairment of the aqueous producing cells or whether the effect was produced indirectly by a receptor-mediated change in blood supply to the ciliary body or reduction of ultrafiltration in the ciliary body.

If, however, the specific β-adrenolytic active component as illustrated is indeed of decisive importance with regard to the antiglaucomatous effect of β-receptor blocking agents, then those β-blocking agents which combine a high, specific β-adrenolytic potency and a non-disturbed local absorption and diffusion to the site of the receptor would surely be most suitable. How does metipranolol fit in here?

When considering the binding affinity of metipranolol to the β-adrenergic receptor, it must be borne in mind that because of its ester structure metipranolol is rapidly decomposed to desacetyl-metipranolol in the tissue. In oral application this decomposition occurs so rapidly and quantitatively that no parent substance whatsoever can be detected in the plasma, but only the metabolite [27]. Fig. 4 illustrates this decomposition process.

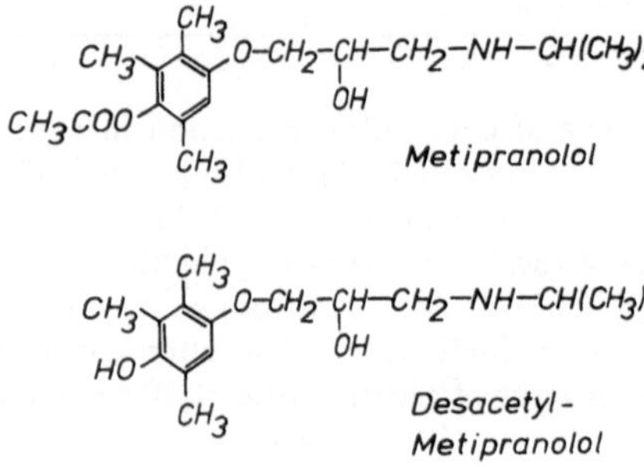

Fig. 4. Structural formulae of metipranolol and its main metabolite desactetyl-metipranolol

We must, therefore, assume that also in the topical use of metipranolol it is not metipranolol but its metabolite which produces the actual pharmacodynamic effect. Because of this we must also take its affinity data into consideration.

In cats under pentobarbital anaesthesia Zakhari et al. [28] determined the shift to the right of the dose-effect curve which is obtained from the increase in heart rate caused by increasing concentrations of isoproterenol. In this manner they obtained pA$_2$ values for the half-maximum occupation of the cardiac β_1-receptors of 8.17 for metipranolol and 8.03 for the desacetyl derivative.

If one compares these date with those of other β-receptor blocking agents used therapeutically [28—32], it is seen that both compounds possess a medium-strong affinity to the β-receptor which more or less corresponds to that of oxprenolol ($pA_2 = 8.12$) and alprenolol ($pA_2 = 8.10$). Table 1 provides a comparison.

Table 1. *pA₂-values of beta-receptor blocking agents as measurement for the half-maximal occupation of cardiac β_1-receptors*

Name of Beta-receptor blocker	pA₂-value for the β_1-receptor
Metipranolol	8.17
Desacetyl-Metipranolol	8.03
Oxprenolol	8.12
Alprenolol	8.10
Bupranolol	9.20
Timolol	8.70
Acebutolol	6.95
Propranolol	8.10

Therefore, on a molar basis metipranolol and its metabolite are weaker in action only by the factor 1.8 and 2.5 respectively as against the standard substance propranolol and by 3.4 and 4.7 as against timolol. The absolute height of this specific beta-adreno-lytic active component, however, should not be decisive for the practical use of the one or the other beta-receptor blocking agent as substances with low affinity, e. g. practolol ($pA_2 = 6.9$ [30]) also have an antiglaucomatous effect when the dose is increased correspondingly.

An additional property of some beta-receptor blocking agents worth mentioning in this connection concerns the so-called cardio-selectivity. This describes the particular property of β-receptor blocking agents, e. g. cebutolol, atenolol, metoprolol, bunitrolol or practolol to interact in preference with the cardiac β_1-receptors. This property can achieve therapeutic importance when patients with airways pulmonary diseases or asthma bronchiale have to be given simultaneous antiglaucomatous treatment.

The cardioselective properties do not seem to have any clear influence directed at the mechanism of reducing intraocular pressure. In experiments on the rabbit eye [7] it was seen that the relatively β_1-selective practolol is particularly effective but there are several other studies which came to contrary conclusions [9, 25, 33]. Metipranolol and its main metabolite adopt a neutral position in that

they like bupranolol and timolol do not belong to the non-selective
β-receptor blocking agents.

Also the so-called intrinsic sympathomimetic activity (ISA) of
some β-receptor blocking agents seems to be of little if any importance for the mechanism of reduction in intraocular pressure. If at
all, this active component would rather exercise a negative effect
[7, 34]. By ISA the property (e. g. of pindolol, alprenolol and aceto-
butolol) is meant that there is not only an antagonistic effect on the
β-receptor but also, in part, an agonistic effect at the same time. In
the rat Bartsch *et al.* [35] confirmed Trčka's results [36] according to
which metipranolol has no frequency increasing intrinsic action and
thus no ISA whatsoever. Clinical findings by Pentikäinen *et al.* [27]
and Hopf *et al.* [37] speak in favour of this.

The physico-chemical properties are beyond doubt of great practical importance for the local penetration and tolerance of β-receptor blocking agents. On its way to the interior of the eye, the drug,
upon local application to the surface of the eye, must first permeate
the cornea in order to reach the vitreous humour. The epithelium,
however, seems to be the most important structure controlling permeability, as, upon its being removed, both fat-soluble and fat-
insoluble substances can readily penetrate the cornea. If, however,
the epithelium is intact, the speed of permeation increases parallel
to the lipophilia of the drug [39]. Again the latter should not be
too pronounced as the drug must also dissolve to a satisfactory
extent in the aqueous humour. Metipranolol and its metabolite
fulfil these prerequisites in an ideal manner as their lipophilia
takes a medium position with values of 4.0 and 3.8 respectively
(determination in chloroform/phosphate buffer) [28]. This is comparable with that of timolol (distribution coefficient octanol/water
= 2.10 [17]). Katz [8] and Schmitt *et al.* [40] demonstrated high
timolol levels in the aqueous humour upon topical use.

Nevertheless penetration studies with the relatively hydrophilic
atenolol [41] and sotalol [7] showed that — also from the theoretic
point of view — unfavourable solubility properties of a β-receptor
blocking agent do not present any absolute obstacle with regard
to reaching the site of action. Rather they influence the onset and
duration of action on the eye. The degree of lipophilia of a β-receptor blocking agent is still of practical-therapeutical relevance in that
such important properties as the membrane-stabilizing cardio-
depressive and local-anaesthetic action correlates direct with this
[42]. In other words conclusions with regard to local tolerance may
be drawn from the lipophilic properties. In our own studies we
determined the distribution coefficient of some relevant β-receptor

blocking agents in comparison to metipranolol in a *n*-octanol-phosphate buffer (pH 7.40)-mixture. The results are given in Table 2.

Table 2. *Distribution coefficients of beta-receptor blockers as relative measure for their lipophilia*

Name of the Beta-receptor blocker	Octanol/Phosphate buffer distribution coefficient
Metipranolol	0.88
Bupranolol	2.88
Propranolol	9.24

From this it is seen that, because its character is much more hydrophilic than bupranolol and propranolol, metipranolol should posses negligible surface anaesthetic activity qualities and this explains the good local tolerance in topical application in contrast to propranolol.

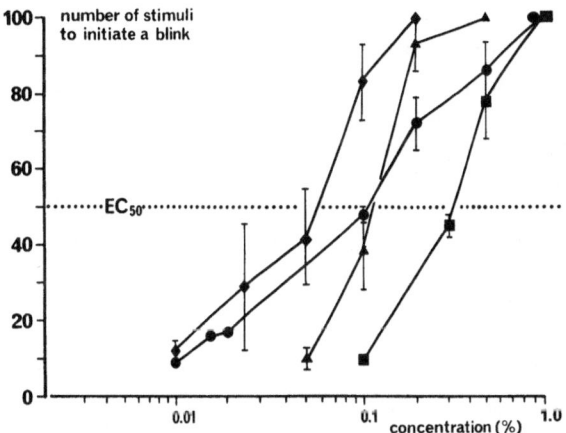

Fig. 5. Examination of surface anaesthesia in the rabbit cornea. $\bar{x} \pm s_{\bar{x}}$, from $n = 6$. EC$_{50}$-values: ▲ Cocaine 0.11 %; ◆ Propranolol 0.06 %; • Pindolol 0.12 %; Metipranolol 0.32 %. (From Bartsch *et al.*, 1977 [35])

Bartsch *et al.* [35] studied the surface anaesthetic properties in the rabbit eye. Fig. 5 shows the results in the form of dose response curves in comparison to cocaine, propranolol and pindolol.

If one takes the effect of propranolol as being equal to 1, metipranolol possesses only one fifth of this action. On account of its lipophilia being almost identical to metipranolol a comparably favourable relationship should apply to the metabolite desacetylmetipranolol.

Summing up we can state that metipranolol and its main metabolite desacetyl-metipranolol are β-receptor blocking agents exhibiting medium β-adrenolytic potency. They are non-cardioselective in effect and do not possess any intrinsic sympathomimetic activity. The relatively slight degree of lipophilia guarantees good absorbent properties without there being negative effects on local tolerance from the surface-anaesthetic active component running parallel to this.

As one must always reckon with a systemic effect in topical application, the same contraindications apply to metipranolol as to all other β-receptor blocking agents when given orally. All in all, the pharmacological active qualities speak for the good suitability of metipranolol for antiglaucomatous therapy.

References

1. Phillips, C. I., Howitt, G., Rowlands, D. J.: Propranolol as ocular hypotensive agent. Brit. J. Ophthalmol. 51, 222—226 (1967).
2. Wettrell, K., Pandolfi, M.: Propranolol vs. acetazolamide. A long-term double masked study of the effect on intraocular pressure and blood pressure. Arch. Ophthalmol. 97, 280—283 (1979).
3. McDonald, M., et al.: Comparison of ocular hypotensive effects of acetazolamide and atenolol. Br. J. Ophthalmol. 61, 345—348 (1977).
4. Elliot, M. H., Cullen, P. M., Philipps, C. I.: Ocular hypotensive effect of atenolol — tenormin I. C. I. — a new beta-adrenergic blocker. Br. J. Ophthalmol. 59, 296 (1975).
5. Bucci, M. G., Missiroli, A., Giraldi, J.: Local administration of propranolol in the treatment of glaucoma. Boll. Oculist. 47, 51—60 (1968).
6. Ros, F. E., Dake, C. L., Nagelkerke, N. J. D., Greve, E. L.: Metoprolol eye drops in the treatment of glaucoma. A double-blind single dose trial of a $beta_1$-adrenergic blocking drug. Graefes Arch. Klin. Exp. Ophthalmol. 206, 247—254 (1978).
7. Bonomi, L., Perfetti, S., Noya, E., Bellucci, R., Massa, F.: Comparison of the effect of nine beta-adrenergic blocking agents on intraocular pressure in rabbits. Graefes Arch. Klin. Exp. Ophthalmol. 210, 1—8 (1979).
8. Katz, I. M.: Beta-blockers and the eye. An overview. Ann. Ophthalmol. 10, 847—850 (1978).

9. Leydhecker, W.: Sympathikomimetika and Sympathikolytika in der Glaukomtherapie. Klin. Mbl. Augenheilk. *171*, 538—546 (1977).

10. Nielsen, N. V.: Timolol und Metoprolol. Okulärer hypotensiver Effekt, lokale und systemische Begleiteffekte. Z. prakt. Augenheilk. *2*, 71—77 (1981).

11. Krieglstein, G. K., Leydhecker, W.: Medikamentöse Glaukomtherapie. München: Bergmann. 1982.

12. Kern, R.: Zur Verteilung der adrenergen Rezeptoren im M. sphincter pupillae, im M. dilatator pupillae und im Ziliarkörper des Menschen; deren Bedeutung bei der Behandlung der Hypotonia bulbi und des Glaukoms. In: Medikamentöse Glaukomtherapie (Krieglstein, G. K., Leydhecker, W., eds.), pp. 133 ff. München: Bergmann. 1982.

13. Sears, M. L., Barany, E. H.: Outflow resistance and adrenergic mechanisms. Effects of sympathectomy, N-(2-chloroethyl)dibenzylamine hydrochloride (dibenamine), and dichloroisoproterenol on the outflow resistance of the rabbit eye. Arch. Ophthalmol. *64*, 839—848 (1960).

14. Takase, M.: Effects of propranolol on aqueous dynamics in primary openangle glaucoma. Acta Soc. Ophthalmol. Jpn. *80*, 310—314 (1976).

15. Potter, D. E.: Adrenergic pharmacology of aqueous humor dynamics. Pharmacol. Review *33*, 133—153 (1981).

16. Vareilles, P., Lotti, V. J.: Effect of timolol on aqueous humor dynamics in the rabbit. Ophthalmic Res. *13*, 72—79 (1981).

17. Cruickshank, J. M.: The clinical importance of cardioselectivity and lipophilicity in beta blockers. Am. Heart J. *100*, 160—178 (1980).

18. Takats, I., Szilvassy, I., Kerek, A.: Intraocularer Druck und Kammerwasserzirkulationsuntersuchungen an Kaninchenaugen nach intravenöser Verabreichung von Propranolol (Inderal). Graefes Arch. Klin. Exp. Ophthalmol. *185*, 331—342 (1972).

19. Öhrström, A., Kättström, Ö.: Interaction of timolol and adrenaline. Br. J. Ophthalmol. *65*, 53—55 (1981).

20. Innemee, H. C., De Jonge, A., Van Meel, J. C. A., Timmermanns, P. B. M., Von Zwieten, P. A.: The effect of selective α_1- and α_2-adrenoceptor stimulation on intraocular pressure in the conscious rabbit. Naunyn-Schmiedebergs Arch. Pharmacol. *316*, 294 298 (1981).

21. Neufeld, A. H., Page, E. D.: In vitro determination of the ability of drugs to bind to adrenergic receptors. Invest. Ophthalmol. Visual Sci. *16*, 1118—1124 (1977).

22. Mittag, T., Tormay, A.: Adrenergic receptors in iris-ciliary body: direct ligand binding studies. Invest. Ophthalmol. Visual Sci. (A. R. V. O. suppl.) *20*, 198 (1981).

23. Dafna, Z., Lahav, M., Melamad, E.: Localization of beta-adrenoceptors in the anterior segment of the albino rabbit eye using a fluorescent analog of propranolol. Exp. Eye Res. *29*, 327—330 (1979).

24. Bromberg, B. B., Gregory, D. S., Sears, M. L.: Beta-adrenergic receptors in ciliary processes of the rabbit. Invest. Ophthalmol. Visual Sci. 19, 203—207 (1980).

25. Nathanson, J. A.: Effects of a potent and specific β_2-adrenoceptor antagonist on intraocular pressure. Br. J. Pharmacol. 73, 91—100 (1981).

26. Thomas, J. V.: Ocular adrenergic receptor sites pertinent to aqueous humor dynamics. Ann. Ophthalmol. 12, 96—98 (1980).

27. Pentikäinen, P. J., Neuvonen, P. J., Penttila, A.: Assessment of beta-blocking activity of trimepranol in man. Int. J. Clin. Pharmacol. 6, 279—284 (1978).

28. Zakhari, S., Pronay, N., Drimal, J., Molnar, L.: Correlations between the partition coefficient and the beta-adrenolytic activities of trimepranol and its analogues. Bratislavské lékařske Listy 62, 678—688 (1974).

29. Bieth, N., Rouot, B., Schwartz, J., Velly, J.: Comparison of pharmacological and binding assays for ten β-adrenoceptor blocking agents and two β-adrenoceptor agonists. Br. J. Pharmacol. 68, 563—569 (1980).

30. Dreyer, A. C., Offermeier, J.: In vitro assessment of the selectivities of various beta-adrenergic blocking agents. Life Sci. 27, 2087—2098 (1980).

31. Kaumann, A. J., McInerny, T. K., Gilmour, D. P., Blinks, J. R.: Comparative assessment of β-adrenoceptor blocking agents as simple competitive agonists in isolated heart muscle. Naunyn-Schmiedebergs Arch. Pharmacol. 311, 219—236 (1980).

32. Noack, E.: Untersuchungen zur spezifischen adrenolytischen und unspezifisch kardiodepressiven Wirkung des β-Rezeptorenblockers Acebutolol. Arzneim.-Forsch./Drug Res. 31, 1410—1416 (1981).

33. Colasanti, B. K., Trotter, R. R.: Effects of selective beta$_1$- and beta$_2$-adrenoceptor agonists and antagonists on intraocular pressure in the cat. Invest. Ophthalmol. Visual Sci. 20, 69—76 (1981).

34. Demmler, N.: Beta-Rezeptorenblocker in der Ophthalmologie. Med. Mo. Pharm. 3, 174—179 (1980).

35. Bartsch, W., Sponer, G., Dietmann, K.: Experiments in animals on the pharmacological effects of metipranolol in comparison with propranolol and pindolol. Arzneim.-Forsch./Drug Res. 27, 2319—2322 (1977).

36. Trčka, V.: Pharmacological activtities of trimepranol and its fate in the organism, Part 2. Res. Institute for Pharmacy and Biochem., Prague 1973.

37. Hopf, R., Tourbier, H., Kaltenbach, M.: Wirksamkeit des Beta-Sympathikolytikums Methypranolol auf Belastungsherzfrequenz und ischämische ST-Senkung im Vergleich mit Plazebo und Propranolol. Herz/Kreislauf 9, 560—565 (1977).

38. Cocan, D. G., Hirsch, E. D.: The cornea, VII. Permeability to weak electrolytes. Arch. Pharmacol. 32, 276—282 (1944).

39. Swan, K. C., White, N. G.: Corneal permeability, I. Sectors effecting penetration of drugs into the cornea. Am. J. Ophthalmol. *25,* 1043—1058 (1942).

40. Schmitt, C. J., Lotti, V. J., Le Duarce, J. C.: Penetration of timolol into the rabbit eye. Measurement after ocular installation and intravenous injection. Arch. Ophthalmol. *98,* 547—551 (1980).

41. Ross, F. E., Innemee, H. C., Van Zwieten, P. A.: Penetration of atenolol in the rabbit eye. Graefes Arch. Klin. Exp. Ophthalmol. *208,* 235—240 (1978).

42. Hellenbrecht, D., Lemmer, B., Wiethold, G., *et al.*: Measurement of hydrophobicity, surface activity, local anaesthesis and myocardial conduction velocity as quantitative parameters of the non-specific membrane affinity of nine β-adrenergic blocking agents. Naunyn-Schmiedebergs Arch. Pharmacol. *277,* 211—226 (1973).

Author's address: Prof. Dr. E. A. Noack, Institut für Pharmakologie, Universität Düsseldorf, Moorenstrasse 5, D-4000 Düsseldorf 1, Federal Republic of Germany.

The Toxicology of Metipranolol with Particular Regard to the Eye

W. Sterner

IBR Forschungs GmbH, Walsrode, Federal Republic of Germany

When applications are made for the registration of drugs containing new substances, sufficient data on experimental toxicological studies must also be submitted. These form the basis for weighing expected benefits against possible hazards, i. e. they should allow decisions to be made concerning the safety of drugs.

The content and volume of such studies must be dependent on the nature of the active ingredient, the indications, the duration of use and the patient population.

Table 1. *Toxicological test program — metipranolol*

I. Acute toxicity

Acute toxicity oral — mouse
Acute toxicity oral — rat
Acute toxicity i. p. — mouse
Acute toxicity i. p. — rat

A toxicological test program was carried out for metipranolol, a non-selective beta-receptor blocking agent for use in glaucoma therapy, and this was accepted by the German Federal Health Board (BGA) as a sufficient basis to weight benefits against risks.

In essence the test program comprised of five major investigation divisions and each one involved a series of individual studies.

Table 2

II. Chronic toxicity

Study with oral application

Study	Object	Dosage (mg/kg)
3 months tox. rat	syst. tox.	0, 20, 100
6 months tox. rat	syst. tox.	0, 5, 20, 100
3 months tox. dog	syst. tox.	0, 25
6 months tox. dog	syst. tox.	0, 5, 25, 75
6 months tox. rat	ocular tolerance	0, 25

Test with topical use		Application
6 months tox. rabbit	ocular tolerance	1 drop of metipranolol 0.6% instilled twice daily into conjunctival sac of both eyes

Table 3

III. Reproduction toxicology
   Reprotox. — rat
   Reprotox. — rabbit

IV. Mutagenicity
   Ames test (with/without metabol. activation Salmonella typh.)
   Sister chromatid exchange (bone marrow Chinese hamster)
   Host-mediated assay (mouse, Salmonella typh., Serratia marescens)

V. Cancerogenicity
   24 months feeding study — rat
   Dosages (mg/kg feeding); 0.275, 550, 1100

Results

With regard to the illustration of results and to make these more understandable, the main aspect of the individual test systems will first be commented upon. Then there will be a summary and assessment of the results.

I. Acute Toxicity

This establishes the toxic effects that a substance causes when it is administered in a *single* dosage.

The best known parameter for the test for acute toxicity is the so-called LD_{50}. This means the quantity of substance, generally expressed in mg or ml/kg body weight, at which, on average, 50% mortalities occur.

Table 4. *Acute toxicity — task and purpose*

Establishment of dose — effect ratio

Recognition of specific toxic action

Assessment of mode of toxicity

Basis for comparison with similar substances

Basis for establishing therapeutic countermeasures in cases of accidental poisoning

Table 5

LD_{50} (with confidence limits)

Species	Application	LD_{50} mg/kg 24 h and 14 days
Mouse	per oral (p. o.)	604.5 (542.9—679.5)
Rat	p. o.	1544.7 (1389.5—1756.3)
Mouse	intraperitoneal (i. p.)	265.4 (258.4—272.7)
Rat	i. p.	239.0 (210.3—277.0)

From these data it can be seen that the LD_{50} of metipranolol is undoubtedly within the range of values corresponding to comparative preparations.

The acute-toxic *target symptoms* of metipranolol were disorders of balance, apathy and tonic cramps. In essence, these are based on the non-specific concomitant phenomena of β-receptor blocking agents.

II. Investigation of Tolerance in Long-term Use

One of the most important studies with drugs is the investigation of tolerance in long-term (chronic) use.

Table 6. *Chronic toxicity*

Investigation of the toxic effect of a substance upon *repeated* use

(Parameters: Clinical studies, blood pressure, ECG, haematology, clinical chemistry, macroscopic, microscopic pathology)

Determination of the "no effect" dose

Investigation of the biological mode of action of toxicity (e. g. cumulation, target organs)

Test for reversibility

Table 7. *Results — rat, rabbit*

A) Emphasis on systemic toxicity

Study	Dose (mg/kg)	Findings
3 months tox. rat	100	fatty degeneration of the liver (low-grade)
6 months tox. rat	5	"no effect" dose
	20 } 100 }	dose-related leucopenia
	100	significantly reduced heart frequency, PQ/QRS intervals prolonged (cardio-depressive action)

Table 8

B) Emphysis on ocular tolerance

Study	Dose (mg/kg)	Findings
6 months tox. rat	20	"no effect" dose
6 months tox. rabbit	1 drop metipranolol 0.6% in both eyes twice daily	"no effect" dose

The following special examinations were carried out on the eyes:

Table 9. *Special eye examination*

	Rat	Rabbit
Draize test [2]		
(cornea, iris, conjunctiva)	+	+
Ophthalmoscopy		
(cornea, anterior chamber, fundus)	+	+
Slit lamp examination		
(cornea, anterior chamber, lens)	+	+
tonometry	−	+
Schirmer test	−	+
Histopathology		
eyes including N. opticus	+	+
upper/lower lid	+	+
retrobulbar tissue	+	+

The following findings were made in dogs (see Table 10).

Table 10. *Results — dogs*

Test	Dose (mg/kg)	Findings
3 months tox.	25	no changes due to test compound
6 months tox.	5	"no effect" dose
	25	loss in weight muscular tremor, vomiting, sedation
	75	loss in weight tremor, ton. cramps, salivation death 5/6 animals
	general	slowing down of heart rate prolongation of PQ and QT segments. Retarding of atrioventricular transmission with a tendency to irregular A.-V. blockade (quinidine-like, cardio-depressive antiarrhythmic action on heart, typical for β-receptor blocking agents)

The deviations from normal findings observed in the chronic toxicity studies are in the main to be accounted for by the pharmacodynamic intrinsic action of the product and must be interpreted in relation to the clinical dose. The maximum daily dose of metipranolol 0.6 % is 1 drop per eye twice daily (20 drops = 1 ml).

Accordingly, 0.01—0.02 mg/kg (depending on body weight) would be administered daily to the patient. As against this there is a clear "no effect" dose in the rat and dog of 5 mg/kg body weight, i. e. the safety limit is 250—500. This range is absolutely adequate, even on the assumption that the total quantity administered is completely absorbed.

The good *local* tolerance established in the long-term studies is in conformity with the studies by Brewitt and Dausch [1], who, after applying metipranolol (twice daily 0.6 %) for five months to the rabbit eye, could not establish any damage to the cornea even by means of scanning electron microscopy.

III. *Establishing the Teratogenic and Embryotoxic Potential*

An important issue in judging the safety of a new drug is establishing its teratogenic and embryotoxic potential.

Table 11. *Reproduction toxicology*

Establishing the embryotoxic/teratogenic influence of a substance on the developing embryo and foetus

Establishing the activity on the post-natal period up to the end of the lactation period (21st day)

Parameters: implantations, absorptions,
                 numbers and weights of foetuses, abnormalities
                 development in weight during lactation
                 number of weanings

The increased number of absorptions in the treatment groups could have been caused by changes in the blood flow (vasoconstriction) in the uterus region.

Table 12. *Reproduction toxicology — results*

Study	Dose per mg/kg	Duration of application	Findings
Reprotox. rat	20 100	1.—19.	nad nad
Reprotox. rabbit	10 20 50	1.—27.	increased number of absorptions

IV. Studies on the Influence of Substances on the Genotype Body Structures

In recent times studies on the influence of substances on the genotype body structures have been proving to be of increasing necessity.

Table 13. *Mutagenicity studies*

Mutagenic effects are irreversible (such as cancerogenicity and teratogenicity)	
The test system must indicate:	
Point mutations	(Ames test with Salmonella typh., host-mediated assay)
Chromosome mutations	Sister-Chromatid-Exchange-Test (SCE test)

Table 14. *Mutagenicity — results*

Study	Dosage	Findings
Ames test (5 Salmonella typh. strains without/with liver homogenate)	5 1—5000 μg/plate	no point-mutagenic activity
Host-mediated assay mouse Salmonella typh.	60 and 200 mg/kg p. o.	no point-mutagenic activity
Serratia marescens		slight mutagenic activity
SCE test (bone marrow Chinese hamster)	1 × 1000 mg/kg p. o.	no chromosomal activity

The results of the test profile exclude, with a great degree of reliability, the probability of a mutagenic effect in humans. A slight mutagenic effect was seen in the host-mediated assay with Serratia marescens a 21 (Leu⁻), but this was accompanied by just as slight an antibacterial effect. From the fact that no antibacterial and mutagenic effect could be detected either in the Ames test (with five test strains S. typhim.) or in the host-mediated assay (with S. typhim. G 46), it is to be concluded that the activities observed with Serratia marescens must be specific to the test organism.

V. Study on Tumorigenic Effects

A study on tumorigenic effects, particularly carcinogenic effects must be carried out in the following instances:

a) Chemical relationship of test substances or its metabolites with known tumorigenic drugs.

b) Any indication of possible tumorigenic effects from chronic studies (e. g. non-inflammatory proliferative changes).

c) Any indications of possible mutagenic effects from in-vitro/in-vivo studies.

d) Long-term use in patients.

Cancerogenic studies are mostly carried out in rats and mice, whereby basically the administration of the test substance covers the *complete* life time. The major parameters include:

Survival rate, number of tumors, occurrence of tumors, type of tumors (particularly benign, malignant).

In these very complex studies the test groups are first of all compared with "actual" control carried out at the same time. Furthermore the findings and data of the so-called "historic control", (i. e. the spontaneous tumor rates, for example) of the animal in the test is taken into consideration when interpreting the experimental findings.

At the moment only an interim report (from the 97th test week) is available on the results of this study.

A slight inhibition in the development of the body weight of the animals in all dose groups was seen but there were no indications of any neoplastigenic properties.

This statement, however, is only to be considered as a tendency as the full period of the study, has not elapsed and, more important, the results of the histological investigations are not yet available.

Summary

On the basis of the results of the toxicological test program one may sum up as follows:

In all phases of the experimental study metipranolol has proved both systemically and locally to be extremely well tolerated.

Thus the product fulfils the high norms laid down for the safety of drugs. However, the result of the cancerogenity study will have to be included in any final decision on the safety of metipranolol.

References

1. Brewitt, H., Dausch, D.: Untersuchungen zur Morphologie des Hornhautepithels nach Langzeitanwendung antiglaucomatöser Augentropfen. Vortrag, 79. DOC-Zusammenkunft, Heidelberg, 1981.
2. Draize, J. H.: Appraisal of the safety of chemicals in foods, drugs and cosmetics. In: Dermal toxicity, pp. 49—51. Kansas: The Association of Food and Drug Officials of the United States. 1959.

Author's address: Dr. Dr. W. Sterner, IBR Forschungs GmbH, Südkampen 31, D-3030 Walsrode 2, Federal Republic of Germany.

Principles of Clinical Drug Trials

G. K. Krieglstein

University Eye Clinic Würzburg
(Director: Prof. Dr. Dr. h. c. W. Leydhecker),
Federal Republic of Germany

The introduction of a new drug often raises the justified question about the procedure to which a chemically defined active compound is submitted before it is available as a commercial product to the medical profession. In view of the updated rules governing the safety of drugs this is indeed a costly procedure and so it is not surprising that only one out of about 6,000 to 10,000 synthetisised substances is approved as a drug for clinical use. In many cases the complete development period may take up to ten years and the costs may be in the range of 80 million DM.

The preclinical studies, which I will only mention briefly, are mainly based on standardized pharmacological and toxicological studies in acute tests and in chronic application, whereby, above all, questions regarding carcinogenicity, teratogenicity, mutagenicity, the influences on fertility and perinatal mortality should be examined.

The quality of drug preparations is regulated in the guide-lines of the German Pharmacopoeia (8th edition). In particular this refers to the identification of the active compound, its purity and content as well as its stability at given temperatures. The evidence of efficacy is based on controlled clinical trials. The safety for use is obtained from the therapeutic index, that is the relation between action and side effects, whereby in individual cases provisions should always be made for the doctor's judgement. The approval of any drug depends ultimately just as much on the pharmacological-toxicological studies as on the clinical studies. Expert opinions on the various sections are submitted to an expert committee which then has to make the decision regarding the licensing.

According to a general pharmacological principle that "a drug is safe when its side effects are acceptable", experience has shown that an effective drug is never free of side effects, whereby these may be acute, have cumulative character, appear only in certain patients, occur in association with other drugs or even be part of the therapeutic effect. The clinical control of drugs is normally divided into four phases.

Phase I is concerned with the preliminary control and first administration to healthy volunteers. It should provide conclusive results on pharmacokinetics (absorption, metabolism, biliary excretion, renal elimination, interaction with other drugs) and bioavailability. Conclusions regarding tolerance and dosage are important for further clinical studies.

Phase II of the clinical evaluation is required to be carried out in the form of a controlled clinical trial. The information expected from phase II is concerned particularly with the efficacy and the optimum dosage in patients, the comparison with a placebo or standard therapy, the compliance or acceptance of the drug by the patient. The controlled study which was formerly also known as the double-blind study, eliminates wishful hoping on the part of the therapeutist or the patient in judging the effect of the drug. The efficacy obtained should be significantly greater than the placebo effects. In many test institutions the basic question as to whether the controlled clinical trial may be too exacting is governed by an ethics commission.

Phase III is concerned mainly with providing information on long-term tolerance and registering side effects which could not be found in the limited studies of phase I and II. The phase III studies are mostly multi-center studies, frequently not controlled and in the main epicritical or retrospective. The volume of results obtained in phase III is frequently not commensurate with the great effort put into the underlying multi-center study but it does provide a greater likelihood of ascertaining rare side effects.

The aim of *phase IV* is to reveal rare but nevertheless important side effects. It may be that the active ingredient was or was not marketed subject to special release conditions and this requires particular vigilance on the part of the doctor.

The repetition of various trials and chance allotment, i.e. randomisation, are amongst the most important principles of biometric test planning. Thus in the case of those parameters which are easily checked, e.g. intraocular pressure, the doctor will not rely on a single measurement and relate efficacy to this but, mindful of the biological variability of the parameter, he will carry out several measurements in order to define the untreated level as accurately as possible. Randomisation mostly takes place by means of a list selected by a computer and this establishes which treatment the volunteer will receive (active compound or placebo) or, in the case of an intra-individual comparison, which eye is given a standard therapy and which the test therapy.

When laying out the test design emphasis will be placed on particular characteristics, e. g. stadium of the disease, certain forms of the disease or certain age groups. A symmetric test set-up is also of importance, i. e. the registering of parameters in terms of time for all groups at the same time.

The test protocol should contain clearly formulated questions and leave no doubt as to the criteria for the inclusion or exclusion of patients. The observation should be carried out in such a manner that as far as possible an exact comparison may be made between the different therapeutic groups. The period of observation or the number of test units may be varied. If, for example, after a short period treatment it is obvious that the test product is superior to the standard therapy, the duration of observation may be shorter than was originally intended in the test design. The ever controversial placebo test remains justified as the most relevant results can still be obtained in the controlled placebo test. It is of great significance to the investigating physician that placebos despite their lacking biological-chemical efficacy can cause a therapeutic effectiveness as well as undesired side effects.

It is one of the volunteer's rights to be informed that he may be allotted to a placebo or true product group. A prerequisite is, of course, that a placebo effect may occur in the particular disease. The disease may not be so severe that the risk of failure in placebo therapy is out of proportion to the advantages of the actual therapy. The course of placebo therapy has to be observed closely and if there is any deterioration in the disease the placebo must be discontinued.

The volunteer should be enlightened on the nature, significance and scope of the clinical trial and in particular he should be informed about the risks involved.

The less experience made with the new drug the more detailed the information should be and a written record should be kept. The Declaration of Helsinki requires that in any research on human beings each potential subject must be adequately informed of the aims, methods, anticipated benefits and potential hazards of the study and the discomfort it may entail. He or she should be informed that he or she is at liberty to abstain from participation in the study and that he or she is free to withdraw his or her consent to participation at any time.

Only when all of these principles have been fulfilled conscientiously by all persons participating in the development of the drug can the degree of safety that the patient expects from the medicamentous therapy of his disease be achieved.

References

1. Ballintine, E. J.: Objective measurements and the doublemasked procedure. Amer. J. Ophthalmol. *79*, 763—767 (1975).
2. Bearman, J. E.: Writing the protocol for a clinical trial. Amer. J. Ophthalmol. *79*, 775—778 (1975).
3. Chalmers, T. C.: Ethical aspects of clinical trials. Amer. J. Ophthalmol. *79*, 753—758 (1975).
4. Davis, M. D.: Application of the princicples of clinical trials. Amer. J. Ophthalmol. *79*, 779—785 (1975).
5. Domschke, S., Domschke, W.: Arzneimittelprüfung heute. Fortschr. Med. *99*, 814—818 (1981).
6. Ederer, F.: Why do we need controls? Why do we need to randomize? Amer. J. Ophthalmol. *79*, 758—762 (1975).
7. Fink, H.: Grundsätze des kontrollierten Versuchs. Arzneim.-Forsch./ Drug Res. *28*, 2017—2019 (1978).
8. Gross, R.: Notwendigkeit und Zulässigkeit der kontrollierten klinischen Prüfung. DÄ *16*, 1091—1100 (1979).
9. Hartmann, E.: Nicht-randomisierte Therapiestudien. Arzneim.-Forsch./ Drug Res. *28*, 2027—2032 (1978).
10. Herman, Z. S.: The principles of controlled clinical trials of drugs. Int. J. clin. Pharmacol. *16*, 361—364 (1978).
11. Kahn, A. H., Leibowitz, H., Ganley, J. P., Kini, M., Colton, T., Nickerson, R., Dawber, R.: Standardizing diagnostic procedures. Amer. J. Ophthalmol. *79*, 768—775 (1975).
12. Kohlhaas, M.: Rechtliche Probleme der klinischen Pharmakologie und Therapie. In: Klinische Pharmakologie und Pharmakotherapie (Kuemmerle, H. P., Garrett, E. R., Spitzy, K. H., eds.), 3rd ed. München — Berlin—Wien: Urban & Schwarzenberg. 1976.
13. Kupfer, C.: The role of clinical drug trial methodology with respect to studies of new drugs. Clinical trials of timolol. Surv. Ophthalmol. *23*, 399—401 (1979).
14. McMahon, G. F.: The effects of new federal regulation on clinical investigation. Clin. Pharmacol. Ther. *23*, 495—496 (1978).
15. Probst, M., Fabian, W.: Zur Durchführung von prospektiven kontrollierten randomisierten Studien in der Klinik. Fortschr. Med. *98*, 1—14 (1980).

16. Remington, R. C.: Problems of university-based scientists associated with clinical trials. Clin. Pharmacol. Ther. *25*, 662—665 (1979).
17. Sommer, A.: Epidemiology and statistics for the ophthalmologist, pp. 1—86. New York: Oxford University Press. 1980.
18. Wolf, G. K.: Probleme in der Anwendung statistischer Methoden bei Therapiestudien. Fortschr. Med. *99*, 803—823 (1981).

Author's address: Prof. Dr. G. K. Krieglstein, Universitäts-Augenklinik, Josef-Schneider-Strasse 11, D-8700 Würzburg, Federal Republic of Germany.

The Local Anaesthetic Action of Metipranolol Versus Timolol in Patients with Healthy Eyes

J. Draeger and R. Winter

University Eye Clinic, Hamburg
(Director: Prof. Dr. J. Draeger),
Federal Republic of Germany

With 4 Figures

In the last few years the topical use of beta-receptor blocking agents to reduce intraocular pressure has gained ground considerably. Wide usage of the first products of this type was, however, hampered by the local anaesthetic side effect on the cornea, as beta-receptor blocking agents have a chemical structure that is similar to that of local anaesthetics. This also partly explains their membrane-stabilizing activity. As far back as 1972 Vale *et al.*, when using propranolol topically, described this unexpected side effect, i. e. a topical anaesthesia of the cornea. The classical type of anaesthetics with a topical action is composed of

1. a secondary or tertiary amino group,

2. a polar carboxy oxygen that may belong to an ester or acid amide and

3. an apolar ring.

The anaesthetising activity is dependent on that portion of the free base which is released in the tissue. We can see a similar structure in almost all beta-receptor blocking agents.

Accordingly, an anaesthetising effect of these substances, in particular of the formerly used propranolol and bupranolol, has been known for some time (Vale *et al.*, 1972; Krieglstein *et al.*, 1977).

We also were able to demonstrate the extent and temporal course
of this local anaesthetic effect in an earlier study with propranolol
and bupranolol.

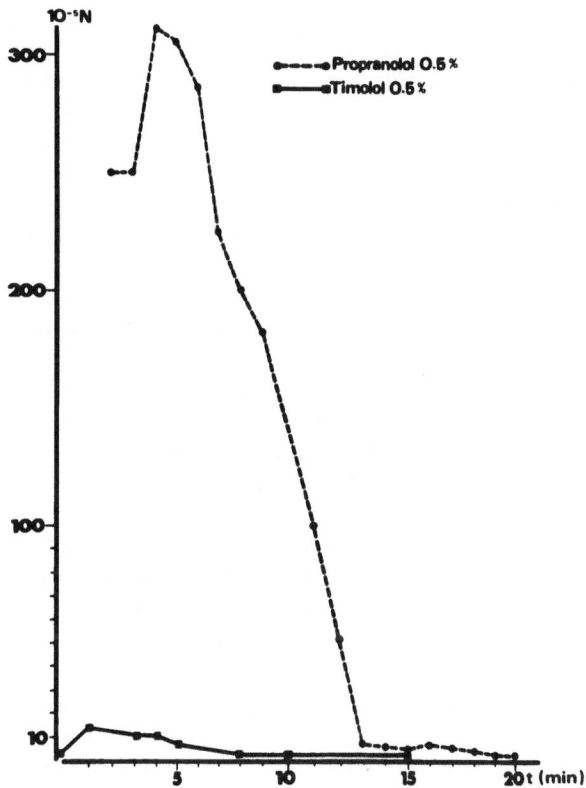

Fig. 1. Local anaesthetic effect of timolol versus propranolol

Upon the introduction of timolol this side effect receded into the
background. This substances proved itself to be particularly well
tolerated. The local anaesthetic action of timolol is much less than
that of propranolol and bupranolol.

Now with metipranolol we have a similarly good substance with
regard to tolerance and pressure reducing action and, therefore,
metipranolol should be compared with timolol with regard to its
local anaesthetic side effect (Fig. 1).

By means of a new electronic optical aesthesiometer we have been in a position for some years now to carry out a sensitivity measurement on the cornea which is truly reproducible quantitatively (Draeger et al., 1976). Environmental parameters (von Frey, 1894) which used to prove disturbing are no longer of significance.

Apart from the precise measurement of irritability an optical control of contact between the measuring instrument and the corneal surface is possible. Place and time of the measurement can be fixed exactly. A rapid automatic approach of the feeler to the corneal surface at a defined speed makes it possible for us to disregard a ballistic effect. The handling of the instrument is very easy and can be done by auxiliary members of the staff (Fig. 2). The measuring apparatus itself is composed of the bent end of a lever arm with a diameter of 0.5 mm.

The force exerted can be read off within a range of 0.1 to $1,000 \cdot 10^{-5}$ Newtons. The place and time when the feeler comes into contact with the cornea can be observed both in the upwards and side view by means of a microscope built into the instrument.

In order to judge any change in sensitivity, it is first necessary to know the normal sensitivity of the cornea. For this reason the topography of the sensitivity thresholds of the cornea was established. Compared to the region near the limbus the corneal centre proved to be particularly sensitive. Even with our method of measuring, the absolute sensitivity threshold of the cornea cannot be established in the healthy eye as, even at the minimum possible force of irritation of $1.0 \cdot 10^{-5}$ N, a supraliminal irritation is still exerted.

However, not only the site of the sensitivity measurement but also age plays a rôle in the sensitivity thresholds. The corneal sensitivity decreases to a very slight but measurable extent in advancing age.

In an earlier study (Buhr-Unger et al., 1980) compared the local anaesthetic effect of propranolol, bupranolol and timolol and it was seen that, as far as sensitivity disorders are concerned, timolol has the slightest side effects. Thus it seemed reasonable to compare the action of metipranolol with that of timolol.

Timolol, a non-selective beta-blocker, has gained ground very rapidly in the treatment of glaucoma (Zimmermann, 1977; Nielsen, 1978; Krieglstein, 1978). Metipranolol, likewise a non-cardioselective beta-blocker, which has been used successfully for some years in the treatment of hypertension, angina pectoris, cardiac dysrhythmia and hyperthyreosis, has very recently become available for local application in ophthalmology. Krieglstein (1982), Mertz (1982),

Bleckmann (1982), von Denffer (1982), Kruse (1982), and Dausch (1982) have reported in detail about the pressure reducing effect of metipranolol applied locally. The therapeutically interesting concentrations seem to be 0.25 % and 1 %.

We have now studied the local anaesthetic effect of metipranolol in concentrations of 0.25 % and 1 % versus timolol 0.25 %. In a randomised double-blind study we tested 20 healthy eyes. Furthermore we are able to include a comparison with timolol 0.5 % from an earlier study.

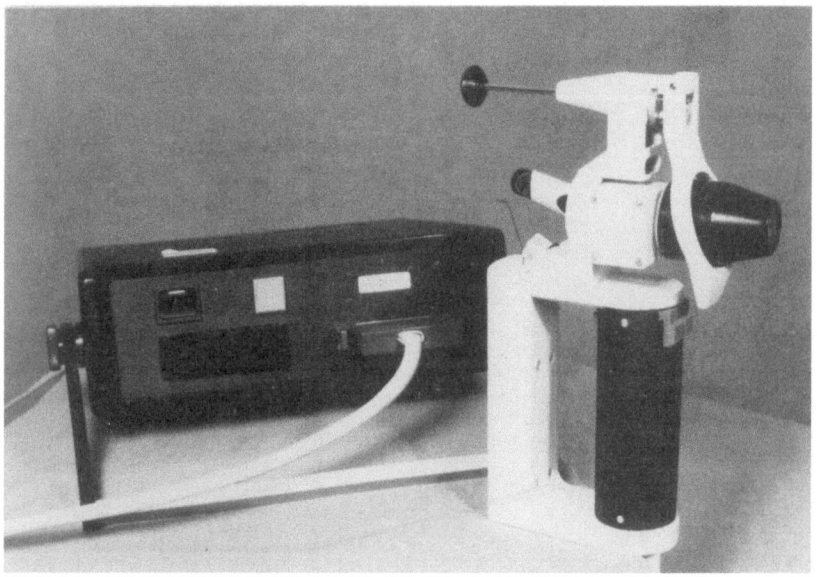

Fig. 2. Portable aesthesiometer with control desk

The age of the patients was between 19 and 60 years, whereby more than half was older than 40 years. All three batches were instilled at random sequence in the same eye of each patient, whereby neither the patient nor the investigator knew the sequence. The interval between applications was not less than 6 hours.

Measurements were carried out with the electronic-optical aesthesiometer in the following manner: the threshold value in the centre of the cornea was determined before the study began and at 6 h.

J. Draeger and R. Winter:

Subsequently we applied 20 μl of the batch in question with an Eppendorf pipette. The threshold value for the corneal sensitivity was determined again after 30 seconds, 1, 3, 10 and 15 minutes.

Results

Measurement in the centre of the cornea proved to be inadequate for a statistical evaluation as the normal threshold values are already so low that irritation with the test method was practically always supraliminal. Therefore any additional slight local anaesthetic action of the beta-receptor blockers tested could no longer be detected with any degree of certainty.

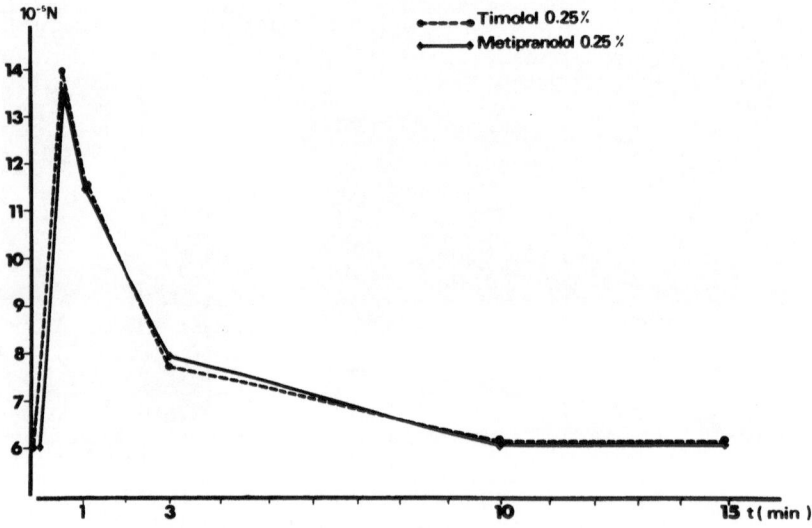

Fig. 3. Mean threshold values and standard deviations after application of metipranolol and timolol 0.25 % at the 6-h-position

The results obtained for each eye and each phase of treatment in the determination of the threshold value at the 6-h-position were considered as the course vector. The differences between measuring courses were evaluated statistically by means of analysis of variance. Immediately upon the application of timolol 0.25 % there was an increase in the threshold value to $13.3 \cdot 10^{-5}$ N and in the case of metipranolol there was an increase from 0.25 % to $13.45 \cdot 10^{-5}$ N. After 10 minutes the initial value was more or less reached again in each case (Fig. 3).

With metipranolol 1 % the threshold value at $12.75 \cdot 10^{-5}$ N reached a similar level as with the 0.25 % solutions. The subsidence rate, however, was clearly slower as was also the case when timolol 0.5 % versus 0.25 % was used (Fig. 4).

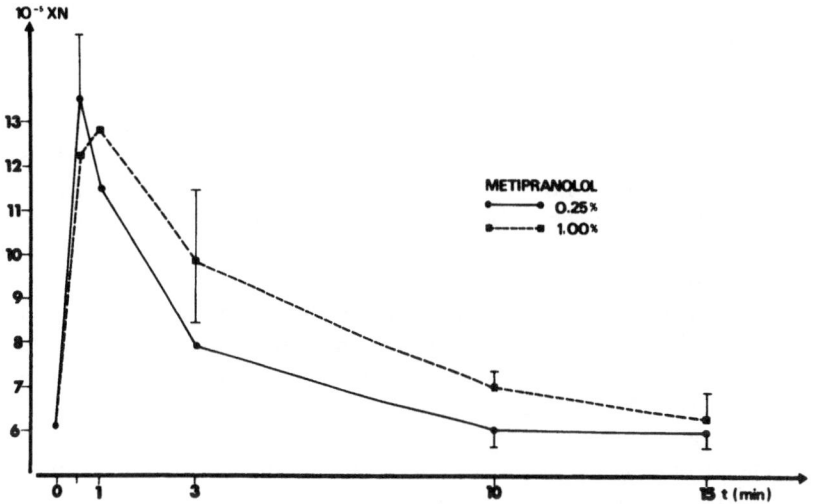

Fig. 4. Course of corneal sensitivity after application of metipranolol 1 % versus 0.25 %

The clearly measurable local anaesthetic effect of all substances could be statistically confirmed in Wilcoxon's preliminary test.

Furthermore, both for metipranolol and timolol, there is a dependency on dose. Any higher dose causes a prolongation in the duration of action between the third and tenth minute after application.

Discussion

The local anaesthetic effect of timolol has already been proved (Buhr-Unger *et al.*, 1980). The series of tests now carried out with timolol and metipranolol confirms this anew. In all beta-receptor blocking agents an almost constant but, all in all, only local anaesthetic effect was observed. The study with two different concentrations of metipranolol shows a direct dependency on dose. The maximum of efficacy is constant but the return to normal sensitivity is delayed with the higher dose. Also in all surface anaesthetics used in ophthalmology we see a curve course which is similar in principle (Draeger et al., 1980).

Because of the slight local anaesthetic effect of timolol and metipranolol no severe damage to the cornea may be expected even in the case of long-term usage. Nevertheless, it should be brought to the patient's notice that after the application of drops a sensation such as that of a foreign body in the cornea could remain unnoticed for some time because of hyposensitivity occurring. For this very reason certain caution is recommended in wearers of contact lenses.

Two other aspects seem to be worth mentioning. First, there are test persons who show a deviating local anaesthetic way of reacting to beta-receptor blocking agents which is genetically determined. In their case there is a significantly higher asensitivity for a longer phase of time.

A damaging effect by beta-blockers might well be possible in such instances. Furthermore, it must be taken into consideration that the studies we are reporting on here were carried out in patients with healthy eyes. A disorder in sensitivity can occur not only in advanced age but also in preceding diseases. For example, in glaucoma we find a reduction in sensitivity related to the duration of the glaucoma. In cases of glaucoma damages with opticus atrophy we find a reduction of corneal sensitivity as compared to a normal group of patients.

As our patients are presenting a very heterogeneous group, it has not yet been possible to prove the data statistically. In the case of a corneal sensitivity primarily already reduced due to previous diseases, such as glaucoma, we are of the opinion that an additional reduction in sensitivity produced by the local application of drugs such as beta-blockers could lead to a damaging decrease in sensitivity.

As we still do not know today to what extent prolonged application might further deteriorate the sensitivity reaction under various circumstances, we are of the opinion that all glaucoma patients under treatment with beta-blockers should be checked from time to time with regard to local anaesthetic side effects. This also applies when such side effects — as is at least the case for timolol and metipranolol — are more or less negligible in patients with healthy eyes.

The statistical evaluation was carried out by Prof. Dr. phil. nat. B. Schneider, Department of Biometry in the Zentrum Biometrie, Medizinische Informatik und Medizintechnik der Medizinischen Hochschule Hannover.

References

1. Bleckmann, H., Pham Duy, T., Grajewski, O.: Therapeutische Wirksamkeit von Metipranolol-AT 0,3 %/Timolol-AT 0,25 %. In: Metipranolol-Symposium. Berlin, 1983. (In this book, pp. 106—120.)

2. Buhr-Unger, H., Draeger, J., Lüders, M.: Untersuchungen zur lokalanästhetischen Wirkung der Beta-Rezeptorenblocker. Ber. Dtsch. Ophthalmol. Ges. *77*, 577—581 (1980).

3. Dausch, D., Brewitt, H., Edelhoff, R.: Metipranolol-Augentropfen — Klinische Verwendbarkeit bei der Behandlung des chronischen Offenwinkelglaukoms. In: Metipranolol-Symposium. Berlin, 1983. (In this book, pp. 132—147.)

4. von Denffer, H.: Wirksamkeit und Verträglichkeit von Metipranolol — Ergebnisse einer multizentrischen Langzeitstudie. In: Metipranolol-Symposium. Berlin, 1983. (In this book, pp. 121—125.)

5. Draeger, J., Koudelka, A., Lubahn, E.: Zur Aesthesiometrie der Hornhaut. Klin. Mbl. Augenheilk. *169*, 407—421 (1976).

6. Draeger, J., Langenbucher, H., Lüders, M., Banner, W.: Zur Wirkung von Oberflächenanaesthetika am Auge. Klin. Mbl. Augenheilk. *177*, 780—788 (1980).

7. Frey, M. von: Beiträge zur Physiologie des Schmerzsinnes. In: Berichte über die Verhandlungen der Königlich-Sächsischen Ges. der Wissenschaften zu Leipzig, Math. Classe. Leipzig: Hirzel. 1894.

8. Krieglstein, G. H.: The intraocular response of glaucomatous eyes to topical applied bupranolol. A pilot study. Graefes Arch. Klin. Exp. Ophthalmol. *202*, 81 (1977).

9. Krieglstein, G. K.: Die Wirkung von Timolol-Augentropfen auf den Augeninnendruck bei Glaucoma simplex. Klin. Mbl. Augenheilk. *172*, 677—685 (1978).

10. Krieglstein, G. K.: Prinzipien klinischer Arzneimittelprüfung. In: Metipranolol-Symposium. Berlin, 1983. (In this book, pp. 71—75.)

11. Kruse, W.: Ergebnisse einer Langzeitstudie mit Metipranolol. In: Metipranolol-Symposium. Berlin, 1983. (In this book, pp. 126—131.)

12. Mertz, M:. Ergebnisse einer multizentrischen Doppelblindprüfung Metipranolol/Timolol über 6 Wochen. In: Metipranolol-Symposium. Berlin, 1983. (In this book, pp. 93—105.)

13. Nielsen, N. V.: Timolol. Hypotensive effect used alone and in combination for treatment of increased intraocular pressure. Acta Ophthalmol. *56*, 504—508 (1978).

14. Vale, J., Gibbs, A., Phillips, C.: Topical propranolol and ocular tension in the human. Brit. J. Ophthalmol. *56*, 770—775 (1972).
15. Zimmermann, T. J., Kaufman, H. E.: Timolol, a beta-adrenergic blocking agent for the treatment of glaucoma. Arch. Ophthalmol. *95*, 601—607 (1977).

Authors' address: Prof. Dr. J. Draeger and Prof. Dr. R. Winter, Universitäts-Augenklinik Hamburg, Martinistrasse 52, D-2000 Hamburg, Federal Republic of Germany.

Pharmaceutical Development of Eye Drops Using the Product Betamann® as an Example

L. Wawretschek

Messrs. Dr. Mann Pharma, Berlin

With 5 Figures

1. Introduction

It is the aim of this paper to provide a brief insight into the problems involved in the pharmaceutical development of an eye drop product, whereby Betamann is used as an example.

The functions of the formulator may be depicted in the following rough schema:

1.1 Finding out the properties peculiar to the active ingredient to be elaborated.

1.2 Establishing the possible pharmaceutical form.

1.3 Optimising the chosen form at the site of application, taking the question of tolerance into particular consideration.

1.4 Finding out a composition with an optimal stability for use and marketing, without influencing tolerance negatively.

2. Carrying Out the Work in Actual Practice

2.1 Finding Out the Properties Peculiar to the Active Ingredient, Whereby Its Reaction in Water Naturally Plays an Important Rôle

The active substance metipranolol presents an organic base which is characterised by the following features:

substituted aromatic residue,
tertiary nitrogen,
isopropanol grouping.

Therefore, the basic structure of a N-alcyl-phenoxy propanol-amine typical for β-receptor blocking agents underlies the molecule.

Name of raw material: metipranolol — mat. no. 3382
Specification (pharmacopoeia): data from manufacturer
Supplier: Messrs. Boehringer/Mannheim
Description: white, crystalline powder without odour

Solubility: readily soluble in alcohol, methanol, chloroform, acetone, dimethyl formamide
very difficult to dissolve in water

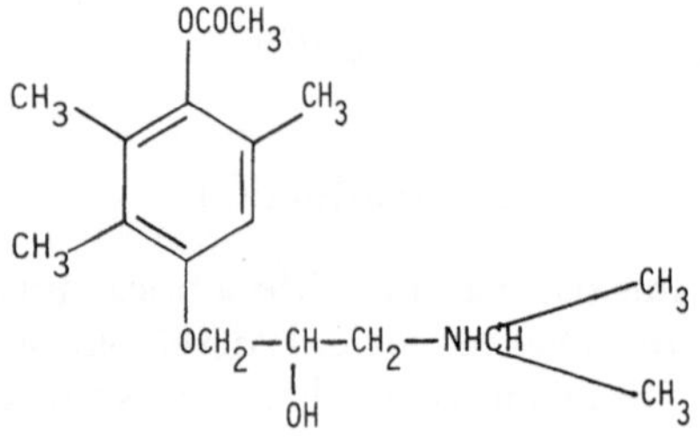

$C_{17}H_{27}NO_4$ mol.-wt.: 309.41

Fig. 1. Properties of active ingredient

The substance is readily soluble in most organic solvents but very difficult to dissolve in water. The presence of tertiary nitrogen, however, improves water solubility to a great extent due to the formation of salt. In the present case the formation of hydrochloride, with which all further examinations were conducted, was chosen from a great number of possibilities. For reasons of time I shall not go into the numerous other properties of the substance which had to be investigated.

2.2 Carrying Out a pH-Screening

After the properties of the substance had been found out, the next step was to carry out a so-called pH-screening in order to find out the optimum pH-value for the future formulation of the actual product.

For this purpose laboratory batches were manufactured in buffered and unbuffered aqueous solution with a concentration of

1 % of the active ingredient. These solutions were subsequently stored in climatic cabinets under stress conditions, i. e. at temperatures of 5, 20, 30, 40 and 50° C.

This type of stress treatment has the advantage that after a relatively short period, i. e. 6 to 12 weeks, a statement can be made on the stability of the active ingredient in relation to temperature.

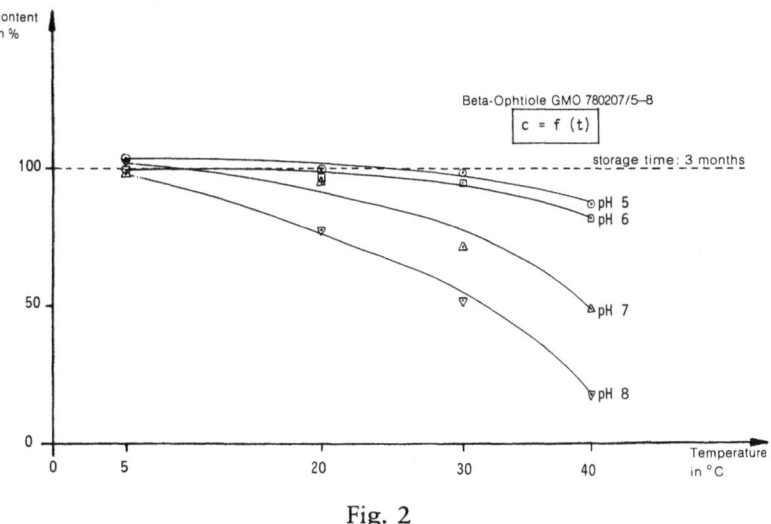

Fig. 2

The Vant Hoff's law of reaction kinetics is used here, whereby the velocity of reaction of a possible decomposition reaction increases between 2 and 4-fold for each 10° C rise in temperature. For the stress test this means that an increase in temperature from 20° C to 50° C results in an increase in the reaction velocity to at least 8-fold. Therefore, after the samples have been stored for 3 months at 50° C, their condition is more or less equivalent to that corresponding to 24 months' storage at room temperature.

After 1.5 and 3 months the solutions are checked as to whether there are any changes in their physical and chemical properties and, in particular, in the concentration of the active ingredient. In order to do this a suitable method of analysis must be worked out. This method must be distinguished by a high selectivity to differentiate the active ingredient from possible decomposition products and by particular sensitivity in order to detect even the slightest changes in the concentration of the active ingredient. Fig. 2 shows the result of this pH-screening after 3 months.

The influence of the pH becomes obvious in the graphic illustration of the dependence of the content of the active ingredient on storage temperature. In our particular case the optimum pH is 5.5 in an unbuffered solution.

Now that these values have been measured, calculations can be made for the predicted stability of the active ingredient at room temperature, whereby two natural laws of reaction kinetics are used. By graphical illustration of the values corresponding to the so-called Arrhenius' equation as $\log k = f(1/T)$, the linearity of this dependence on the decomposition reaction observed is proved.

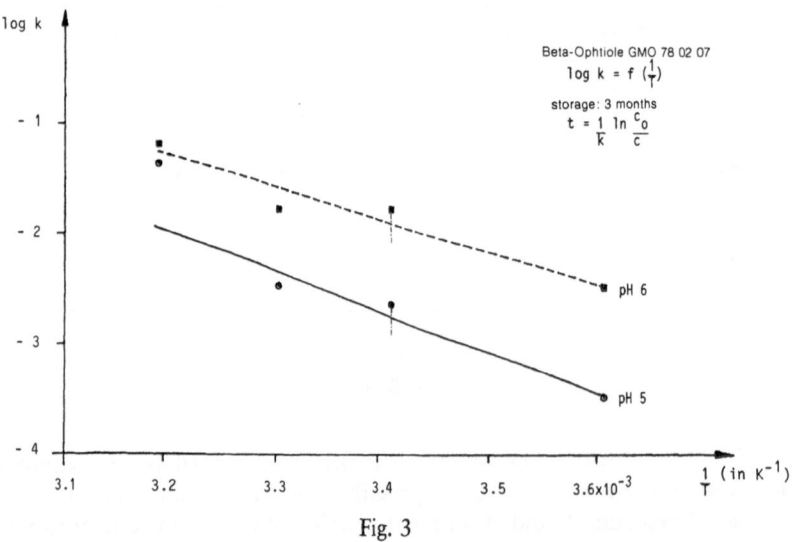

Fig. 3

From this the reaction velocity constants at the range of temperature relevant in actual practice can be calculated and in turn from these, in accordance with the speed-time law of 1st order, the time can be assessed when the concentration falls below the 90% limit stipulated by law. In this manner a stability of more than 3 years at a pH-value of 5.5 could be predicted for the product Beta-Ophtiole.

2.3 Developing Possible Formulations

With the above result the two most vital prerequisites for the development of possible formulations for an aqueous eye drop preparation are given.

When formulating the drug dosage form, the following parameters, which in the main determine the properties of eye drops, are to be observed:

2.3.1 pH

Tolerance:

Physiological value: 7.4
Limits tolerated: 5—11

Biological availability:

Efficacy pilocarpine 0.5% at pH = 6.5 ≙ efficacy
Pilocarpine 4% at pH = 4

2.3.2 Osmotic Pressure

Tolerance:

Physiological value about 290 mOsmol
Limits tolerated: 180—450

2.3.3 Concentration of Active Ingredient

Tolerance:

Substance-specific parameter

2.3.4 Viscosifying Agent

Formation of film:

Increase in adhesive power and retention time on eye
Improvement in absorption (see Fig. 4)

Tolerance:

Improvement by smear effect
Deterioration in non-tolerated substances due to longer retention time

2.3.5 Preservative

Wetting agent:

Better distribution of solution due to decrease in surface tension
Increase in absorption and/or penetration (see Fig. 5)

2.4 Preparation of Test Batches

2.4.1 Manufacture

The next step is the manufacture of various test batches according to the following criteria:

a) Observance of preliminary data from pH-screening
b) Variation of concentration of active ingredient
c) Variation of preservative
d) Variation of viscosifying agent

If one proceeds systematically, the number of batches required may easily exceed a total of 50 and this results in considerable analytic investment.

2.4.2 Storage and Stability Test

After being filled into bottles of various materials, the test batches are stored in climatic cabinets at temperatures of 5^0 to 50^0 C, as was the case with the pH-screening, and their stability is tested at periodic intervals. The complete period of observation is 5 years. The following tests are carried out:

Change in physical properties
Content of active ingredients
Content of preservative and
Development of possible decomposition products

By means of these stress tests the non-stable solutions may be eliminated in many cases after a tested period of 3 months but mostly after 6 months and a selection of the formulations suitable for clinical trials may be made so that, at this stage of testing, the analytical side of the investment has been reduced quite considerably.

From those formulations which have been selected initial samples can now be provided for animal experiments and clinical trials, the particular aim of which is to assess the concentration of the active ingredient and the tolerance. The results of these studies finally lead to the choice of the most favourable composition, with which further extensive clinical trials can then be carried out. During the relatively long period required for these clinical trials, stability tests continue with a small selection of formulations, whereby the results for samples after storage at room temperature are now of decisive

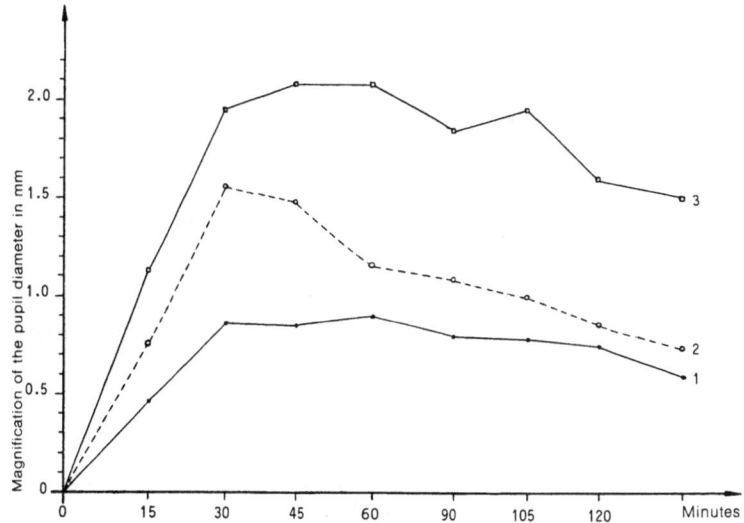

Fig. 4. Influence of viscosity increasing substances on the permeation of homotropine 0.0075 % through the rabbit cornea [Wang, E. S. N., Hammarlund, E. R.: J. Pharm. Sci. 59, 1559 (1970)]

1 aqueous solution, 2 aqueous solution with 1.4 % polyvinyl alcohol (approx. 4 cP), 3 aqueous solution with 0.5 % hydroxypropylmethyl cellulose (approx. 20 cP)

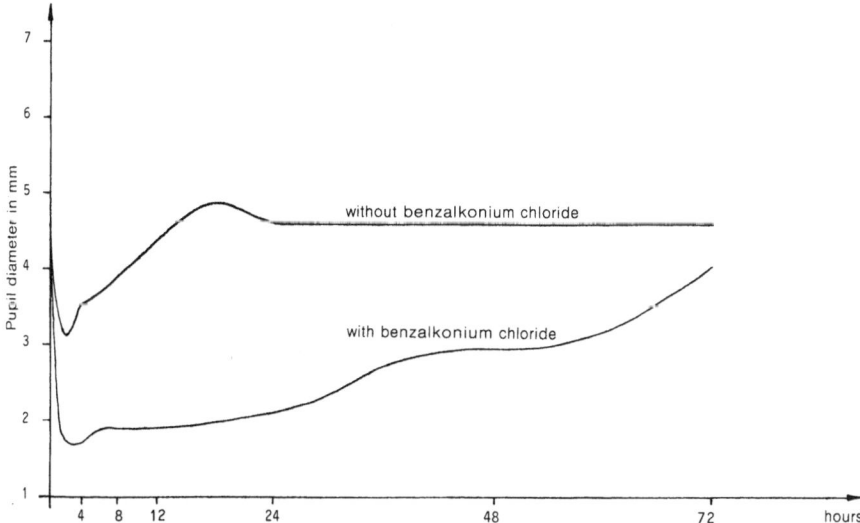

Fig. 5. Influence of benzalkonium chloride 0.03 % on myosis due to carbachol 1.5 % [O'Brien, C. S., Swan, K. C.: Arch. Ophthalmol. 27, 253 (1942)]

importance and, in general, should now prove to be better than those pre-calculated in the stress tests.

In the case of the product Betamann the joint decision of our medicinal-scientific department and the galenics department produced two formulations, the main characteristics of which are as follows:

Concentration of the active ingredient 0.3 % and 0.6 %;

pH 5.5, unbuffered;

benzalkonium chloride as preservative;

polyvinyl pyrrolidone as viscosifying agent and as film-forming agent;

more than 3 years' stability.

Author's address: Dr. L. Wawretschek, Messrs. Dr. Mann Pharma, Brunsbütteler Damm 165-173, D-1000 Berlin 20.

Results of a 6 Weeks' Multicenter Double-blind Trial Metipranolol Versus Timolol

M. Mertz

Eye Infirmary and Outpatient Eye Clinic rechts der Isar —
Technical University, Munich
(Director: Prof. Dr. med. H.-J. Merté),
Federal Republic of Germany

With 4 Figures

1. Introduction

There is already a large number of substances and preparations available for drug therapy in glaucomatous diseases.

Nevertheless, it still seems commendable to develop further drugs as the individual responsiveness with regard to extent and duration of efficacy as well as long-term effectiveness is extremely varied. Apart from the clinical adjustability of intraocular pressure, the conduct of intraocular pressure under normal every day conditions is also of particular interest. The treatment of outpatients in the ophthalmologist's practice affords an ideal opportunity of studying this relationship.

In the following I shall report on a study on the influence of metipranolol on intraocular pressure, whereby circulatory parameters and tolerance were checked at the same time. Subject to regular controls this study was carried out as a double-blind trial in three ophthalmological practices in the Munich area during a total period of 6 months.

2. Materials and Methods

2.1 Trial Set-up

The study was designed as a multi-center cross-over study. It was carried out by three doctors, each of whom treated 9 patients. The treatment was divided into two successive phases of 3 weeks in each case. One group of patients (group 1) was given timolol in the first phase and metipranolol in the second phase. The remaining patients (group 2) were given metipranolol first and timolol subsequently. The allotment into either group was carried out at random and was double-blind, i. e. neither the doctor nor the patient knew in which phase timolol or metipranolol was being administered.

1 drop of a 0.25% solution of each product was instilled twice daily into the eyes. Before the study began the vehicle was applied for 3 days. Thereafter the first phase of treatment lasting 3 weeks began. At the beginning of treatment, after 1 week and after 3 weeks the intraocular pressure of both eyes, blood pressure and pulse rate were determined about the same time of day. Moreover the objective tolerance was determined for the period of treatment just completed and slit lamp findings were made. After the first phase of treatment the doctor presented an overall report on tolerance.

The second phase of treatment was carried out immediately after the first phase. After 4 weeks and at the end of the complete treatment, i. e. 6 weeks, the intraocular pressure of both eyes, blood pressure and pulse rate were measured and the subjective and objective tolerance assessed. At the end the patient was asked whether in his opinion the tolerance of batch A in the first phase of treatment was as good as, better or not so good as batch B in the second phase of treatment. The findings were recorded in the protocol sheets provided, and they form the basis of the statistical evaluation.

2.2 Group of Patients

The study comprised of patients with bilateral chronic glaucomas. Altogether 15 patients were allocated to group 1 (first timolol and then metipranolol); 12 patients were allocated to group 2 (first metipranolol and then timolol). There were 7 male and 18 female patients. No indication of sex was given in the case of 2 patients.

The mean age was 68 years (standard deviation 10 years); the youngest patient was 43 and the oldest 88 years of age.

The intraocular pressure of each patient before any antiglaucomatous treatment was initiated was taken from the doctor's records on the patients. This value served as an initial value in order to calculate any change in the course of the study.

Secondary Findings

Out of the 27 patients 12 had hypertension and 2 suffered from rheumatism. All of the patients except one had already had an antiglaucomatous treatment, whereby timolol had often been used. Treatment was discontinued in good time before the study began.

3. Results

3.1 Changes in Intraocular Pressure

The mean intraocular pressure of the last 3 to 5 measurements prior to initiation of the study as well as the mean values of systolic blood pressure, diastolic blood pressure and pulse are given in Table 1 together with the standard deviations as well as the lowest

Table 1. *Mean starting data at the point of time t (mean values of the last 3 to 5 measurements before and at the beginning of the study)*

	Mean value	Standard deviation	Minimum	Maximum
Intraocular pressure right (mmHg)	22.8	4.7	17	36
Intraocular pressure left (mmHg)	22.4	5.3	16	40
Systolic blood pressure (mmHg) ..	148.3	27.2	115	220
Diastolic blood pressure (mmHg) ..	90.1	10.8	70	110
Pulse (beats/minute) ..	68.8	10.1	50	92

and highest values. The pressure values of both eyes were similar; they showed considerable variability (from 17 to 36 mmHg and from 16 to 40 mmHg).

Table 2. Mean intraocular pressure of patients in the 3 centers of treatment and allocation groups

	n	Before treatment		At the beginning of study		1st phase of treatment				2nd phase of treatment			
						1st week		3rd week		4th week		6th week	
		R	L	R	L	R	L	R	L	R	L	R	L
Doctor 1, Dr. A.													
group 1	3	26.0	23.3	23.0	22.0	19.3	19.0	21.0	19.3	20.7	20.7	22.7	20.3
group 2	5	26.4	24.8	20.0	20.4	21.4	21.4	21.0	21.0	20.6	20.6	19.2	19.0
total	8	26.3	24.3	21.1	21.0	20.6	20.5	21.0	20.4	20.6	20.6	20.5	19.5
Doctor 2, Dr. H.													
group 1	8	28.9	28.9	25.5	25.3	24.1	22.9	22.9	23.0	24.1	24.3	23.8	24.3
group 2	1	28.0	24.0	33.0	30.0	26.0	25.0	26.0	25.0	26.0	23.0	24.0	21.0
total	9	28.8	28.3	26.3	25.8	24.3	23.1	23.2	23.2	24.3	24.1	23.8	23.9
Doctor 3, Dr. K.													
group 1	3	31.3	34.0	17.3	18.0	18.0	19.3	16.7	19.7	16.3	21.0	19.0	19.3
group 2 6	6	25.7	26.3	20.8	20.8	17.3	17.0	17.2	17.3	17.5	16.7	17.8	17.8
total	9	27.6	26.9	19.7	19.9	17.6	17.8	17.1	18.1	17.1	18.1	18.2	18.3

Table 2 shows the mean intraocular pressure values split up according to the centers of treatment and randomised groups.

From this it can be seen that at the beginning of the study the intraocular pressure had already been clearly reduced due to pretreatment.

A summarized illustration of changes in intraocular pressure in the course of the study is given in Table 3 and in Figs. 1 and 2.

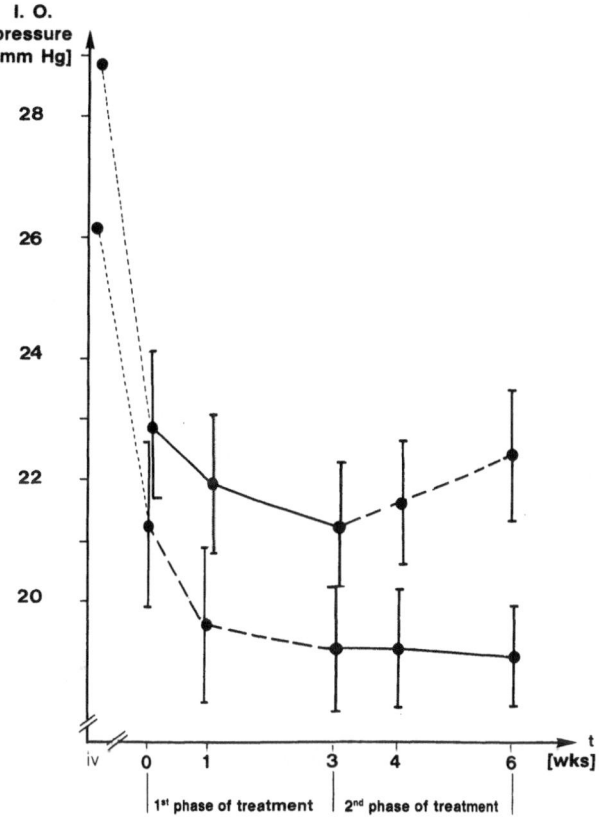

Fig. 1. Behavior in intraocular pressure in the course of the study (in each case in the patient's right eye. Mean values and standard deviations $N = 27$). Clear reduction in pressure due to prior treatment, slight statistically non significant additional reduction during study. - - - - previous treatment, ———— timolol 0.25 % 2× daily, — — — metipranolol 0.25 % 2× daily, iv = initial value, 0 beginning of study

Table 3. Mean values and standard deviations of initial values of intraocular pressure and of the changes as against initial value in the course of the study (in the changes the pooled standard deviation within the center of treatment and allocation groups is given)

| | Before treatment | | Change in intraocular pressure versus initial value | | | | | | | | | |
| | | | Beginning of study | | 1st week | | 3rd week | | 4th week | | 6th week | |
	R	L	R	L	R	L	R	L	R	L	R	L
Group 1 (n=14)					Timolol				Metipranolol			
$\bar{x}$	28.79	28.79	5.57*	5.79*	7.00*	7.50*	7.22*	7.29*	7.07*	6.00*	6.29*	6.43*
s	3.38	6.49	3.08	5.99	2.68	3.92	3.17	4.33	2.70	4.54	4.18	5.16
Group 2 (n=12)					Metipranolol				Timolol			
$\bar{x}$	26.17	25.50	4.67*	4.08*	6.42*	6.00*	6.83*	6.00*	6.67*	6.67*	7.25*	6.92*
s	1.99	1.98	2.45	3.17	3.29	2.37	2.81	2.28	2.53	3.33	3.23	3.06
Total (n=26)												
$\bar{x}$	27.58	27.27	5.15*	5.00*								
s	3.07	5.14	2.81	4.93								

* Change is significantly different from nil ($\alpha < 0.05$).

In Table 3 the mean initial pressure as well as the change in this pressure in the course of the study is given for all centers of treatment. The standard deviation of the change was calculated in each case within the centers of treatment and pooled via the centers, so that it is not influenced by differences between the centers.

A statistical calculation was carried out with the paired t test as to whether the change in the pressure values is statistically significant as against the initial value (before treatment) ($\alpha < 0.05$).

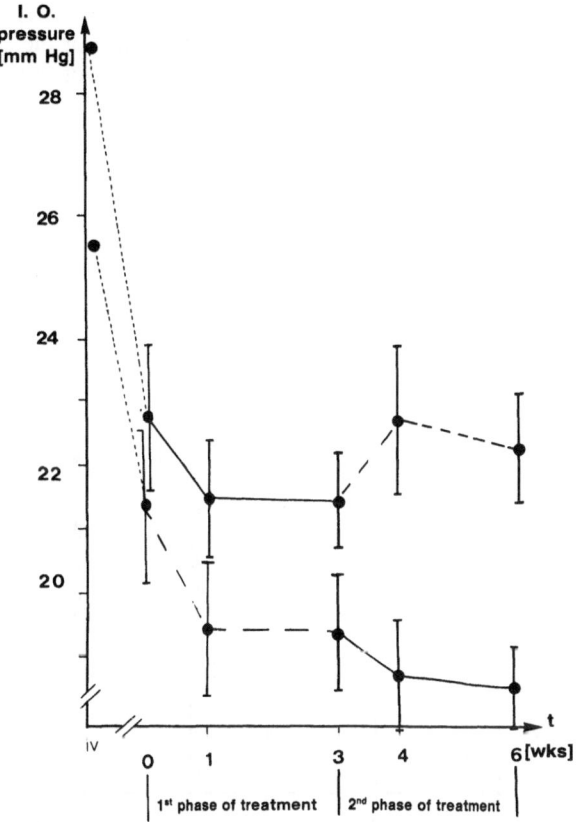

Fig. 2. Behavior of intraocular pressure in the course of the study (referring in each case to the patient's left eye. Mean values and standard deviations $N = 27$). Distinct reduction in pressure due to previous treatment, slight statistically insignificant additional reduction during the study. ---- previous treatment, —— timolol 0.25 % twice daily, – – – metipranolol 0.25 % twice daily, iv = initial value, 0 beginning of study

This is the case for all values (also at the beginning of the study). Table 3 shows that the mean pressure could be reduced further during the course of the study. The difference to the value at the beginning of the study, however, is not statistically significant. Neither is there any significant difference between treatments with timolol and metipranolol.

3.2 Behavior of Blood Pressure and Pulse

The mean values and standard deviations of blood pressure and pulse for the individual measuring times in the study are illustrated in Figs. 3 and 4. Neither the changes in the course of the study nor the differences between the treatments and phases of treatment are statistically significant.

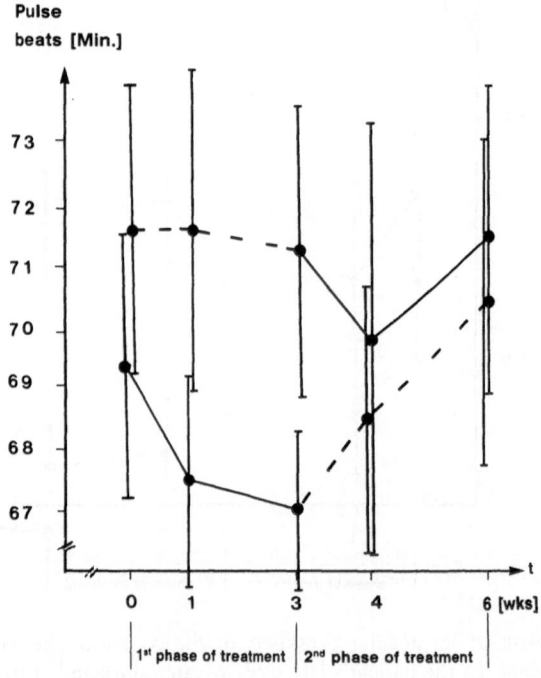

Fig. 3. Behavior of pulse during the study (mean values and standard deviation $N = 27$). No significant influence detectable. —— timolol 0.25 % twice daily, - - - metipranolol 0.25 % twice daily

3.3 Tolerance

The frequency data concerning subjective and objective tolerance are shown in Table 4a (for patients in allocation group 1) and 4b (for patients in allocation group 2).

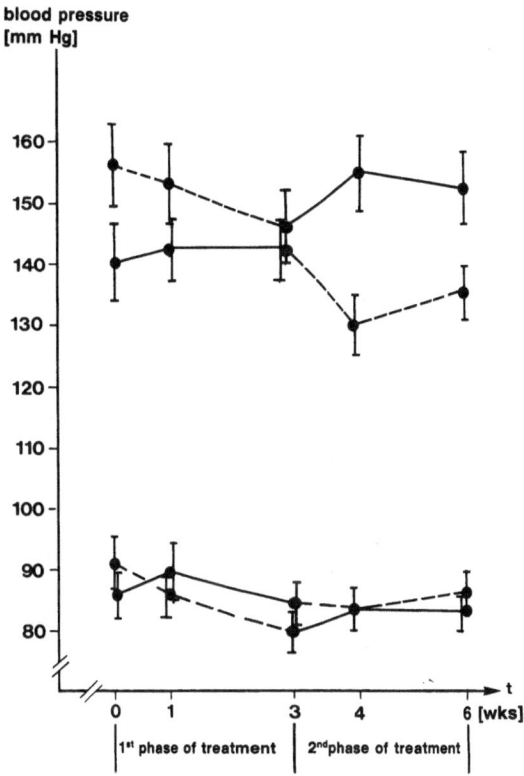

Fig. 4. Behavior of systolic and diastolic blood pressure during the study (mean values and standard deviations $N = 27$). No significant influence detectable. ——— timolol 0.25 % twice daily, – – – metipranolol 0.25 % twice daily

From the tables it is seen that the tolerance of timolol was better than that of metipranolol. During the phase of treatment with timolol stinging was reported only 5 times altogether (at the various times of observation), whereas this was reported altogether 34 times under treatment with metipranolol.

The overall judgement concerning the comfort of timolol was very good in 19 patients, good in 7 patients and satisfactory in 1 patient. Under metipranolol treatment, however, it was very good in 6 patients only, good in 13 patients, satisfactory in 6 patients and not good in 1 patient (for 1 patient no data was given on tolerance in the metipranolol phase).

Table 4 a. *Frequency data on subjective and objective tolerance in the group 1 patients*

Group 1 (Timolol — Metipranolol)

Subjective tolerance

		Neutral	Stinging	Other complaints
T	1st day	14	1	0
	1st week	12	2	2
	3rd week	15	0	0
M	4th week	5	9	1
	6th week	3	11	1

Objective tolerance

		Normal	Allergy	Slit lamp findings without findings	with findings
T	1st day	15	0	15	0
	1st week	15	1	14	1
	3rd week	14	1	14	1
M	4th week	14	1	15	0
	6th week	13	1	12	2

Overall judgement of tolerance after 3 weeks (timolol)
very good: 11   good: 3   satisfactory: 1   not good: 0

Overall judgement of tolerance after 6 weeks (metipranolol)
very good: 2   good: 7   satisfactory: 4   not good: 1

Judgement of patients: batch A (timolol) was
as good as: 6   better than: 5   not so good as: 3

batch B (metipranolol) with regard to comfort.

In the overall judgement of patients concerning tolerance there is, however, no great difference between the two preparations. 11 patients judged both products to be equally good, 5 judged timolol to be better and 3 metipranolol to be better. 3 found timolol to be not so good and 2 metipranolol to be not so good (in 3 patients the comparison of tolerance was not given).

Table 4b. *Frequency data on subjective and objective tolerance in the group 2 patients*

Group 2 (Metipranolol – Timolol)
Subjective Tolerance

		Neutral	Stinging	Other complaints
M	1st day	10	2	0
	1st week	7	5	0
	3rd week	4	7	1
T	4th week	11	1	0
	6th week	11	1	0

Objective tolerance

		Normal	Allergy	Slit lamp findings without findings	with findings
M	1st day	12	0	12	0
	1st week	12	0	12	0
	3rd week	12	0	10	2
T	4th week	12	0	12	0
	6th week	12	0	10	2

Overall judgement of tolerance after 3 weeks (metipranolol)
very good: 11   good: 6   satisfactory: 2   not good: 0

Overall judgement of tolerance after 6 weeks (timolol)
very good: 8   good: 4   satisfactory: 0   not good: 0

Judgement of patients: batch A (metipranolol) was
as good as: 5   better than: 3   not so good as: 2

batch B (timolol) with regard to comfort.

4. Discussion

The present double-blind study metipranolol versus timolol was conducted on glaucoma patients who had already been under ophthalmological treatment for some time. Therefore the previous therapy had already produced a distinct reduction in intraocular pressure from a mean pressure of 27.4 mmHg to 22.4 mmHg, whereby many patients had already been given timolol. After the initiation of the new therapy, the pressure — measured against the mean values — was reduced somewhat again. In the first group it was 20.1 mmHg after the timolol phase and 21.0 mmHg after the subsequent metipranolol phase. In the second group it was 21.0 mmHg after metipranolol and 20.3 mmHg after timolol. At the most it may be said that these results indicate a tendency, as the differences from pressures at the beginning are not statistically significant. On the other hand they do give evidence that the therapeutic use of the new substance metipranolol did not allow any increase in pressure once the previous therapy, which by the large had been effective, was discontinued. In terms of retrogradation, it can, therefore, be considered as being therapeutically safe. Also the differences between patients treated with timolol and metipranolol are not significant and statistically it does not play any rôle whether treatment is first conducted with timolol and then with metipranolol, or vice versa. This shows that, not only with regard to reduction in pressure but also with regard to the dosage scheme and concentration, therapy with metipranolol in this study proved to be remarkably similar to timolol therapy and the results of treatment could not be differentiated statistically.

These results are in conformity with the experience gained recently in a clinical trial with a completely different test set-up (Merté and associates, 1982).

The same can be established for the examined circulatory parameters, blood pressure and pulse. No influence on these parameters could be detected due to treatment.

With regard to tolerance it is noticeable that the detailed statement "stinging more frequent with metipranolol than with timolol" is inconsistent with the overall judgement given by the patients: "comfort more or less equally good with both eye drops". This contradiction cannot be simply disregarded. The most likely explanation is that, all in all, the patients did not attach such a great significance to the "stinging" and it may even be taken as certain that it did not cause them discomfort to any great extent.

It was not necessary in any of the cases to discontinue therapy because of intolerance (either due to the one or the other product).

The statistical evaluation was carried out by Prof. Dr. phil. nat. B. Schneider, Department of Biometry in the Zentrum Biometrie, Medizinische Informatik und Medizintechnik der Medizinischen Hochschule Hannover.

References

Merté, H.-J., Mertz, M., Stryz, J.: Augendruck unter Metipranolol-Einwirkung. In: Medikamentöse Glaukomtherapie (Krieglstein, G. K., Leydhecker, W., eds.), pp. 123—128. München: J. F. Bergmann. 1982.

Author's address: Prof. Dr. M. Mertz, Augenklinik und -poliklinik rechts der Isar der Technischen Universität München, Ismaninger Strasse 22, D-8000 München 80, Federal Republic of Germany.

Therapeutic Efficacy of Metipranolol Eye Drops 0.3% Versus Timolol Eye Drops 0.25%

A Double-blind Cross-over Study

H. Bleckmann, T. Pham Duy, and O. Grajewski

University Eye Clinic, Clinical Center Charlottenburg,
Free University Berlin

With 7 Figures

Since the introduction of β-sympathicolytics in the treatment of elevated intraocular pressure a great number of studies on β-receptor blocking agents dealing with the dynamics of the aqueous humour have been conducted. Ever since the pressure reducing effect was first described in 1970 [1], timolol represents the most widely used β-blocking agent. Timolol is to be classified along with the non-cardioselective β-blocking agents, i. e. responsible for the blockade both at the cardial β-1-receptors and at the extra-cardial β-2-receptors of the bronchi and vessels. The newly developed β-blocking agent metipranolol demonstrates slight β-blocking equipotent doses to inhibit isoproterinol tachycardia compared with propranolol. It exhibits very slight sympathomimetic properties and, measured by the elevation of the fibrillation threshold in electrically stimulated rabbits hearts [2], it shows extremely slight membrane-stabilizing properties. The slight β-stimulating property (intrinsic sympathicomimetic activity) both of metipranolol and timolol as well as their slight cardioselectivity already indicate that both drugs are contraindicated in patients with obstructive airways diseases. Relevant studies on the action of non-cardioselective β-blocking agents with and without this effect on the airway resistance [3] and in patients with small airways disease [4] have already been presented. A first clinical study on the action of metipranolol in glaucomatous eyes was published in 1982 [5]. On the basis of the comparison with timolol with regard to maximum reductions in intraocular pressure after single medication with mean value and calculation of range of diffusion, the authors concluded that the action of metipranolol and timolol on intraocular pressure in glaucoma patients is about equal. Studies are also available on the topical anaesthetising effect of metipranolol on corneal sensitivity [6].

It was the aim of the present study to examine the effect on intraocular pressure with metipranolol 0.3 % in comparison to timolol 0.25 % and do pin down the antiglaucomatous efficacy statistically.

Material and Methods

Altogether 20 patients, 11 of whom were male and 9 female, were examined. The age of the patients was between 27 and 81, the mean age being 69. 6 of the patients exhibited unstable hypertension, none of these patients where given a systemic β-blocker medication. Both eyes of the 20 patients were examined. The iridocorneal angles were of varying width but never narrow. 4 of the patients included in the study had already been pretreated with different concentrations of timolol over a long period. None of the tested patients was aphakic or had undergone an antiglaucomatous operation. The central visual activity was up to 0.5 in 6 eyes, up to 0.7 in 7 eyes and up to 1.0 in 27 eyes. In the determination of the visual field by means of Goldmann perimetry 22 eyes were found to have normal outer limits, 6 eyes showed concentric constriction and paracentral scotomas were detected in 18 eyes. There were 14 incidences of papilla without excavation and 14 eyes showed a flat excavation. 12 eyes were clearly excavated and in none of the cases was any marginal excavation of the papilla found. In 19 patients the clinical diagnosis was glaucoma chronicum simplex and in one patient low tension glaucoma.

The prospective study was conducted in the form of an intraindividual cross-over test. The first 4 days of the study served as a blank phase for all patients. On the 4th day intraocular pressure was determined with the applanation tonometer in the morning, at noon and in the evening and at the same time blood pressure and pulse frequency were measured. The test drug was handed out to the patients on the 4th day and they were instructed to instill 1 drop into both eyes after getting up in the morning and 1 drop into both eyes in the evening. The test phase I lasted from the 5th to the 26th day. On the 1st day of the test tonometry was carried out 3 times and the blood pressure and pulse frequency were determined, as was also the case on the last day of the blank phase. 1 week later both the intraocular pressure and the circulatory parameters were measured once. On the 26th day the intraocular pressure was again measured 3 times and the blood pressure and pulse frequence once. After a blank phase of 4 days test phase II was carried out in the same manner. The initial data of the 3 intraocular pressure measurements used for the statistical calculation refer to an arithmetic mean value. During test phase II two of the patients discontinued the test without giving reasons. The test was conducted after the patients had been enlightened as to its purposes and had given their consent. The eye drops which were applied topically were solutions of metipranolol eye drops 0.3 % and timolol eye drops 0.25 %. The sequence of which product was to be used as the 1st or 2nd drug was established before the test began and was known neither to the investigator nor the patients. The 2 drugs were supplied in identical plastic bottles. Part of the statistical evaluation was carried out by Prof. Dr. B. Schneider, Hanover.

Results

Fig. 1 shows the effect of a 0.3 % metipranolol solution upon single application as the average reduction in pressure for the day in comparison with the blank measurement. The rates of reduction in pressure under metipranolol in phases I and II are illustrated. It is seen that, but for one exception, all eyes demonstrated a pressure sinking effect. According to the values in phase I the reduction in pressure seems to behave in proportion to the initial pressure, i. e. that eyes with high pressure values before treatment experienced a stronger reduction in pressure than those with lower initial values. Metipranolol 0.3 % also reduced intraocular pressure in all eyes on the 1st day of test phase II. Even if the initial pressure of all measurements is lower than in phase I, the pressure sinking effect is to be seen in all eyes without exception.

The pressure sinking effect of metipranolol 0.3 % on the 21st day is illustrated in Fig. 2. 2 eyes in the test phase showed a refractory response in pressure towards metipranolol, whereas the other eyes exhibited a reduced intraocular pressure. In this case also it is seen that the pressure sinking effect at a high initial pressure proves to be greater than in eyes with only a slightly increased pressure. As a rule metipranolol 0.3 % produced an increase in intraocular pressure on the 21st day except for 2 eyes in phase II, i. e. in eyes which had been treated with timolol in phase I.

Correspondingly, Fig. 3 shows the results of a reduction in intra-ocular pressure due to timolol 0.25 % in glaucomatous eyes. The effect on the 1st day in phase I indicates that without exception all eyes demonstrated a decrease in intraocular pressure.

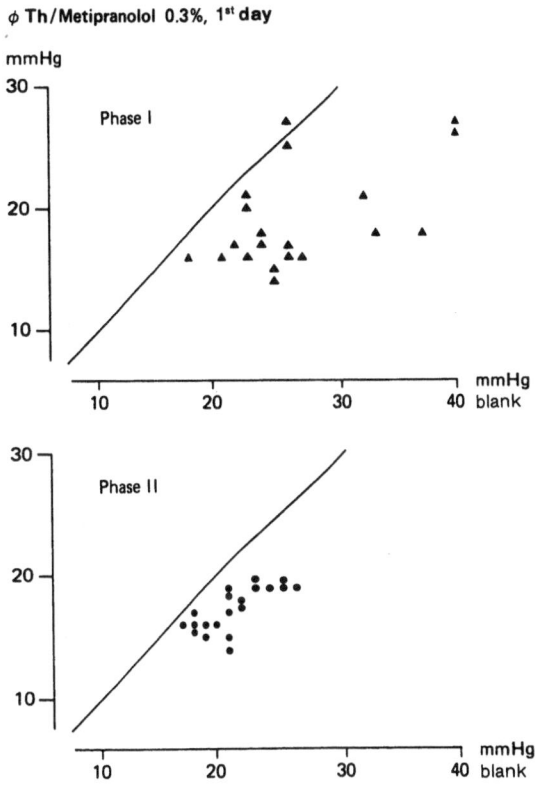

Fig. 1. The effect of metipranolol 0.3 % on intraocular pressure. The effect of treatment on the first day in phase I (above) and phase II (below) is illustrated

Timolol 0.25 % also reduces intraocular pressure on the 1st day of treatment in almost all eyes in test phase II, i. e. in eyes which had already been treated with metipranolol 0.3 %. In this group also there were, however, 2 cases in which the intraocular pressure was not reduced and even increased in comparison to the blank phase.

110   H. Bleckmann, T. Pham Duy, and O. Grajewski:

Fig. 4 demonstrates the pressure sinking effect of timolol eye drops 0.25 % after 21 days. After 3 weeks of treatment it can seen that, when timolol was applied as the 1st drug, upon the determination of intraocular pressure all values were clearly reduced. Timolol 0.25 % in phase II shows a lasting pressure sinking effect except in 2 eyes which did not respond to timolol.

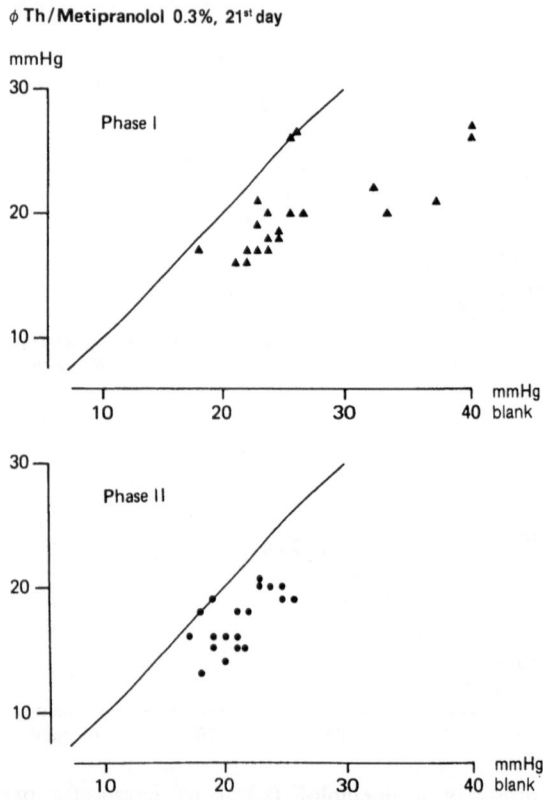

Fig. 2. The action of metipranolol 0.3 % on intraocular pressure after 3 weeks of treatment. The reduction in phase I (above) and phase II (below) is illustrated

The mean values and standard deviations of the daily pressure averages for each measuring point and each phase of treatment are recorded in Fig. 5. From this it is seen that, already on the 1st day both under metipranolol and timolol, intraocular pressure was clearly reduced with a significance of $p < 0.01$ (paired t test). From the temporal course of the treatment it is to be seen that the reduced pressure level was more or less maintained, even though it becomes evident that, as the duration of treatment progresses, the average pressure values of all eyes increased slightly.

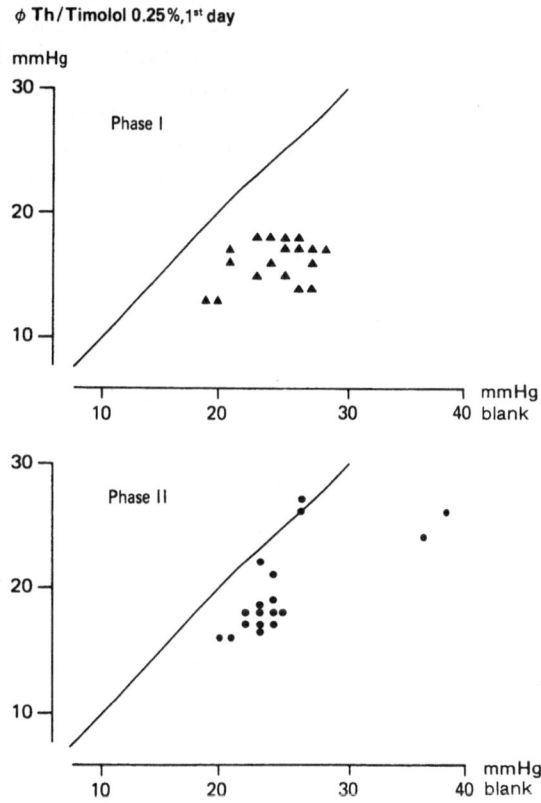

Fig. 3. The effect of timolol 0.25 % on intraocular pressure on the first day of treatment. The effect of reduction in pressure in phase I (above) and phase II (below) is illustrated

One of the reasons for the slight increase is the therapy-refractory conduct of eyes which, independent of the type of medication, became evident in the previous figures. After the blank period at the beginning of the 2nd phase of treatment (day 27 to day 31) the mean pressure values clearly increased again but decreased both under timolol and metipranolol when the 2nd phase of treatment was initiated.

The individual standard deviation of daily fluctuations in intra-ocular pressure was on average between 1 mmHg and 2 mmHg in the course of the complete study and showed no dependence on treatment or phase of treatment.

Table 1 illustrates the difference in intraocular pressure between the mean value before each phase of treatment and the mean value at the end of the phase of treament together with the standard error and the mean percentage of decrease as against the individual value.

The change with the paired t test was checked statistically. Statistically highly significant differences ($p < 0.01$) were obtained for each phase of treatment and each treatment. The difference was between 19 and 27% of the individual value. Table 1 does not

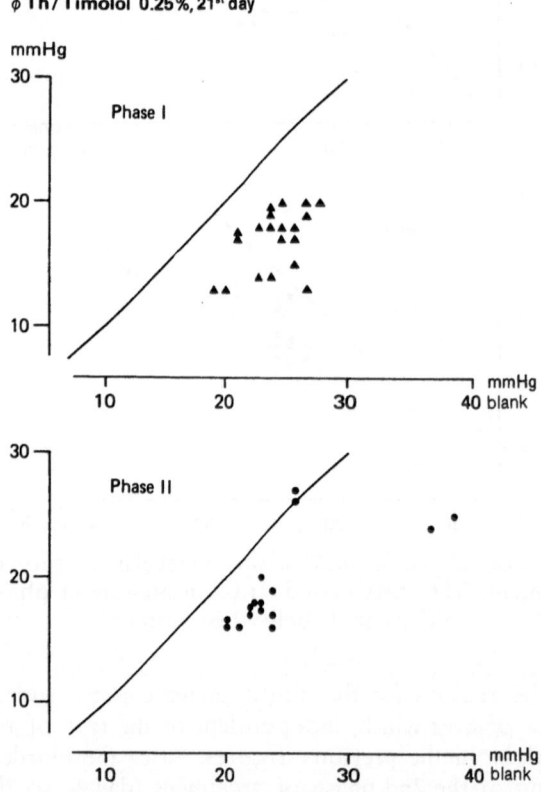

Fig. 4. The effect of timolol 0.25% on intraocular pressure after 3 weeks of treatment. The reduction in pressure in phase I (above) and phase II (below) is illustrated

show any specific differences between treatment with metipranolol and timolol.

In order to examine the influence factors on intraocular pressure more accurately a linear statistical analysis was conducted, whereby

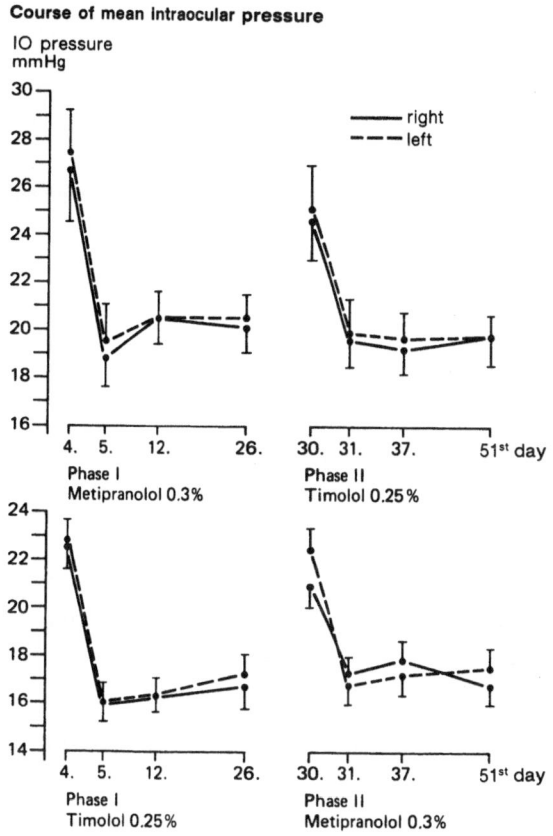

Fig. 5. Mean values and standard deviations of daily pressure averages for metipranolol 0.3 % and timolol 0.25 % under consideration of phase influence in both eyes

the so-called effects which express the influence of the drug (difference between metipranolol and timolol) the phase of treatment (difference between the first and second phase of treatment) as well as the interaction between the drug and phase of treatment were calculated from the measured values (mean daily pressure).

A standard error of mean values calculated to each of the effects and the hypothesis that the relevant effect is 0 was checked with the paired t test. The results are given in Table 2: for the intraocular pressure the drug effect (difference between metipranolol and timolol) is not statistically significant either for the right or the left eye.

Table 1. *Mean change in intraocular pressure in the course of the phases of treatment (separated according to treatments)*

	Phase of treatment I		Phase of treatment II	
	0.3% metipranolol	0.25% timolol	0.3% metipranolol	0.25% timolol
Intraocular pressure right (mmHg)				
mean difference	−6.3*	−6.1*	−4.0*	−5.1*
% of initial value	−24%	−27%	−19%	−20%
standard deviation of mean difference (SEM) .	1.6	0.6	0.6	1.3
Intraocular pressure left (mmHg)				
mean difference	−6.4*	−5.9*	−4.2*	−5.5*
% of initial value	−24%	−26%	−20%	−22%
standard deviation of mean difference (SEM) .	1.3	0.8	0.7	1.3

* The change is statistically highly significant ($p < 0.01$) in the paired t test.

Only for the right intraocular pressure was there a significant phase difference. As can be seen from Table 1 the mean changes in intraocular pressure obtained in the first phase are clearly greater than those obtained in the second phase but no significant interaction between treatment influence and phase influence is given. This means that neither in the first nor in the second phase is there any difference in the change in intraocular pressure obtained with metipranolol and with timolol. In the second phase, however, the reduction in pressure obtained under both drugs is slighter than in the first phase. This can be attributed to the lower initial pressure which as an after-effect of the first treatment was clearly lower at the beginning of the second phase of treatment than at the beginning of the first phase of treatment.

Table 2. *Result of statistical analysis: divided into effect of drug, phase and interaction*

	Effect	Standard error	t
Intraocular pressure right			
medicament	0.424	0.237	1.789
phase	− 0.799	0.237	− 3.371*
interaction	− 0.303	0.732	− 0.414
Intraocular pressure left			
medicament	0.570	0.250	2.280
phase	− 0.486	0.250	1.944
interaction	− 0.345	0.727	0.475

* Statistically the effect is highly significantly different from 0, $p < 0.01$.

If one compares the pressure sinking effect of metipranolol and timolol with each other, this can be illustrated graphically as in Fig. 6 which compares the differences in pressure of both drugs on the first day. It becomes evident that, when metipranolol is used as the first drug (phase I), almost all values are above the diagonals and thus reduce better than timolol. Furthermore, one can see from the figure that all eyes which were treated with timolol as the first drug exhibit the higher decrease in pressure and are therefore plotted under the diagonals. This shows a strict phase dependence of the drugs with regard to their pressure decreasing effect. A numeric counting of the localisations above and below the diagonals clearly demonstrate more comparison points below. This corresponds to a greater effect of timolol. However, in the drawing test this difference is not statistically significant ($p > 0.05$).

Fig. 7 shows a comparison of the pressure sinking effect between metipranolol and timolol on the 21st day of treatment. From this figure it is seen that there is a phase dependence in the reaction of pressure. In Fig. 7 there is also a higher number of comparison points in favour of a reduction in pressure by timolol but in the drawing test no statistical significance ($p > 0.05$) is to be found.

Table 3 gives the mean differences between the initial value before the phase of treatment and the value at the end of the phase of treatment with regard to the conduct of blood pressure and heart frequency. In some instances these parameters rose and in others they fell.

Table 3. *Mean difference in blood pressure and pulse frequency in the course of the phases of treatment (separated according to treatments)*

	Phase of treatment I		Phase of treatment II	
	0.3% metipranolol	0.25% timolol	0.3% metipranolol	0.25% timolol
Blood pressure systolic (mmHg)				
mean difference	+7.2	−1.5	0.0	−2.9
standard deviation	6.8	7.4	3.6	4.7
Blood pressure diastolic (mmHg)				
mean difference	−1.1	−4.0	+5.5	−5.0
standard error	4.6	4.3	3.1	3.6
Heart frequency (beats/minute)				
mean difference	+1.1	−4.0	−4.4	−1.1
standard deviation	2.4	2.8	2.7	1.6

Thus under metipranolol 0.3% a slight increase in the mean difference of the systolic blood pressure is found in phase of treatment I and, under the same drug, an increase in the mean difference of the diastolic pressure is found in phase II of treatment. The mean difference in heart frequency also shows a slight increase in the phase I of treatment under metipranolol but the difference in the compared parameters is not statistically significant ($p > 0.05$) in the paired t test. It can therefore be established that blood pressure and pulse did not change significantly in the course of the phase of treatment.

The frequency data on subjective and objective tolerance are given in Table 4. It is seen that several patients under timolol treatment mentioned stinging: 3 out of 10 patients in the first phase of treatment and 6 out of 10 patients in the second phase of treatment.

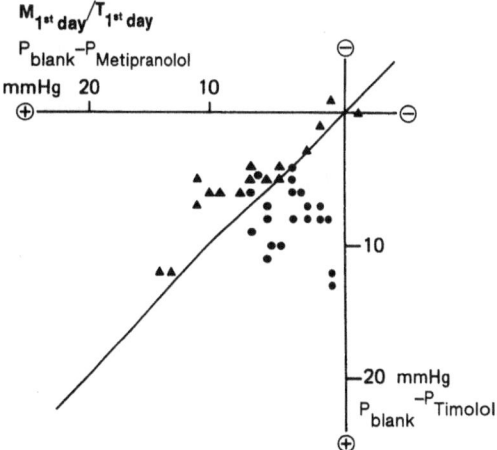

Fig. 6. A comparison of the pressure reducing effect of metipranolol 0.3 % and timolol 0.25 % on the first day does not show any statistically significant difference between the drugs (drawing test $p > 0.05$). ▲ Metipranolol, ● Timolol

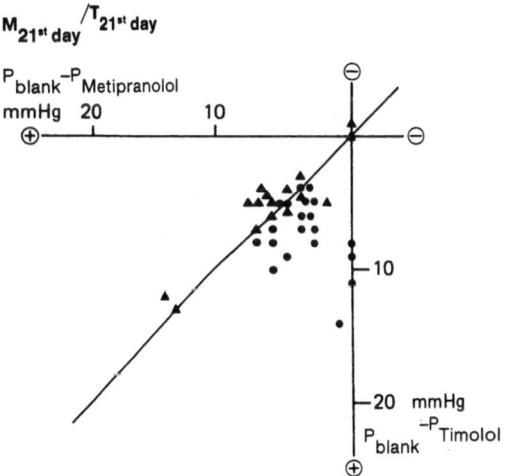

Fig. 7. A comparison of the pressure sinking effect of metipranolol 0.3 % and timolol 0.25 % after 3 weeks of treatment does not show any statistical significant difference between the drugs (drawing test $p > 0.05$). ▲ Metipranolol, ● Timolol

Table 4. *Subjective and objective tolerance of metipranolol 0.3% and timolol 0.25%. 2 patients in group II discontinued treatment after phase I*

	Group I		Group II	
	Phase I metipranolol $n=10$	Phase II timolol $n=8^*$	Phase I timolol $n=10$	Phase II metipranolol $n=10$
Subjective tolerance				
neutral	7	7	9	4
stinging	3	—	1	6
flow of tears ..				(1)
headache				(1)
tiredness				(1)
other complaints		nephelopia (blurring)	(blurred vision)	
Objective tolerance				
normal	10	8	10	9
allergy	—	—	—	1
Overall judgement of tolerance				
very good	1	4	3	—
good	8	5	5	7
satisfactory ...	1	1	2	3

* The changes are not statistically significant ($p=0.05$) in the paired t test.

An allergic reaction was stated by 1 patient only under treatment with metipranolol (in the second phase of treatment). 4 patients claimed that treatment with timolol was more comfortable than that with metipranolol. 13 patiens considered the comfort of both treatments to the equally good and 1 patient as bad. Details are not available for 2 patients as they were excluded from the study earlier.

Discussion

The β-receptor blocking agents metipranolol and timolol under study belong to the non-cardioselective β-sympatholytics and may be used in the treatment of glaucoma. Metipranolol and timolol reduce intraocular pressure on the first day of treatment in phase I by 30 % and 30 % and in phase II by 22 % and 21 %, in relation to the initial pressure. A reduction in pressure in phase I by about 30 % is below the initial reduction in pressure of more than 40 % found hitherto [7] and an adequate explanation cannot be given for this.

The relative. reduction in pressure of metipranolol and timolol on the 21st day in phase I was 24 % and 27 % and these values are in conformity with the results of other investigators [8, 9, 10]. The comparison of both drugs shows a conformity in the relative reduction in intraocular pressure with regard to test phase II: on the first day metipranolol reduced the pressure by 22 % and timolol by 21 %. A corresponding effect is also found after 3 weeks for metipranolol with 20 % and timolol with 21 %. It is to be assumed that the lower initial level which was obtained is due to the pre-treatment. The parameters which have been illustrated do not depict any vital difference between metipranolol and timolol eye drops with regard to their pressure sinking effect in the glaucoma-tous eyes.

β-blocking agents as eye drops can be detected systemically even if only in slight concentrations and can exert an influence on blood pressure and heart frequency as has been reported in 1980 [11]. The decrease in blood pressure and heart frequency can be ex-plained by competitive inhibition from the characterization as non-selective β-blocking agents. A corresponding effect was detected in our study for metipranolol and timolol. In isolated instances the application of metipranolol produced an increase in systolic and diastolic blood pressure and in heart frequency. This effect might best be compared with a slight intrinsic activity on the β-receptors although this property could so far not be proved for metipranolol. In this connection it must be mentioned that all β-blocking agents without proven intrinsic sympathicomimetic activity represent a con-siderable danger for patients with obstructive airways diseases.

The statistical evaluation was carried out by Prof. Dr. phil. nat. B. Schnei-der, Department of Biometry in the Zentrum Biometrie, Medizinische Infor-matik und Medizintechnik der Medizinischen Hochschule Hannover.

References

1. Hall, R., Robin, R. D., Share, N.: A new potent β-adrenergic block agent, 3-morpholine-4-(3-b-butylamine-2-hydroxypropoxy) 1-2-5. thio-diazole hvdrogen maleate. Proc. can. Fed. Biol. Soc. *13*, 33—39 (1970).

2. Bartsch, W., Sponer, G., Dietmann, K.: Experiments in animals on the pharmakological effects of Metipranolol in comparison with Propranolol and Pindolol. Drug Res. *27*, 2247—2426 (1977).

3. Bleckmann, H., Dorow, P.: Die Wirkung von Timolol- und Pindolol-Augentropfen auf den intraokularen Druck und Atemwegswiderstand. In: Medikamentöse Glaukomtherapie (Krieglstein, G. H., Leydhecker, W., eds.), pp. 151—157. München: Bergmann. 1982.

4. Dorow, P., Bleckmann, H.: Die Wirkung von Timolol- und Pindolol-Augentropfen auf die großen und kleinen Atemwege bei Patienten mit einer small-air-ways-disease. In: Medikamentöse Glaukomtherapie (Krieglstein, G. K., Leydhecker, W., eds.), pp. 158—162. München: Bergmann. 1982.

5. Merté, H.-J., Mertz, M., Stryz, J.: Augendruck unter Metipranolol-Einwirkung. In: Medikamentöse Glaukomtherapie (Krieglstein, G. K., Leydhecker, W., eds.), pp. 189—193. München: Bergmann. 1982.

6. Draeger, J., Buhr-Unger, H., Winter, R.: Die Wirkung von Beta-Rezeptoren-Blockern auf die Hornhautsensibilität. In: Medikamentöse Glaukomtherapie (Krieglstein, G. K., Leydhecker, W., eds.), pp. 195—199. München: Bergmann. 1982.

7. Krieglstein, G. K.: Langzeituntersuchung zur augendrucksenkenden Wirkung von Timolol-Augentropfen. Klin. Mbl. Augenheilk. *175*, 627—633 (1979).

8. Radius, R. L., Diamond, G. R., Pollak, K., Langham, M. E.: Timolol — A new drug for management of chronic simple glaucoma. Arch. Ophthalmol. *96*, 1003—1006 (1978).

9. Ritch, R., Hargett, N. A., Podos, S. M.: The effect of 1.5% Timolol — an aleate on intraocular pressure. Acta ophthalmol. *56*, 6—11 (1978).

10. Moss, A. P., Rich, R., Hargett, N. A., Kohn, A. N., Smith, H., Podos, S. M.: A comparison of the effects of Timolol and Epinephrine on intraocular pressure. Am. J. Ophthalmol *86*, 489—495 (1978).

11. Merté, H.-J., Merkle, W.: Timolol-Augentropfen in der Glaukomtherapie. Ergebnisse einer Langzeitstudie. Klin. Mbl. Augenheilk. *177*, 562—571 (1980).

Authors' address: Prof. Dr. H. Bleckmann, Universitäts-Augenklinik des Klinikums Charlottenburg, Freie Universität Berlin, Spandauer Damm 30, D-1000 Berlin.

Efficacy and Tolerance of Metipranolol — Results of a Multi-center Long-term Study

H. von Denffer

Eye Infirmary and Outpatient Eye Clinic rechts der Isar — Technical University, Munich, Federal Republic of Germany

With 1 Figure

Introduction

After the efficacy of metripranolol was clinically established for the first time by Merté *et al.* [4], the question was brought up as to whether a pressure-reducing action similar to other β-blockers might also be observed over a prolonged period and whether metipranolol might, in consequence, prove to be suitable as a reliable pressure-reducing drug for the long-term treatment of open angle glaucoma.

Materials and Methods

In a multi-center study altogether 5 practising ophthalmologists in the region of Munich and Passau tested metipranolol in concentrations of 0.3 or 0.6% during a period of 6 months. Both the intraocular pressure and possible side effects were checked 2 weeks, 2 months and 6 months after the beginning of the study. Altogether 47 patients were included in the study, whereby 44 could be controlled during the complete duration of the study. There were 30 women and 17 men and the mean age was 67.7 years, the youngest patient being 31 and the oldest 85 years of age.

46 patients had open angle glaucoma and 1 patient had a narrow angle glaucoma. 42 patients had already undergone topical antiglaucomatous therapy before the study was initiated, whereby treat-

ment had in the majority of cases been with miotics and not with other beta-blocking agents.

Five of the patients included in the study had a newly diagnosed glaucoma. Metipranolol 0.3% was used in 46 patients and 0.6% initially applied in 1 patient. A change in the dose was necessary in 4 patients on account of unsatisfactory pressure reduction at the low concentration of the drug. Normally the drug was instilled twice daily.

Apart from the subjective and objective tolerance particular attention was paid to the influence of the drug on circulatory functions such as blood pressure and pulse frequency.

Results and Discussion

The efficacy of metipranolol treatment in the course of the test period can be seen in Fig. 1. Before the beginning of therapy with the drug the mean pressure was 27.4 ± 4.2 in the right eye and 27.3 ± 4.1 mmHg in the left eye. These pressure values were taken from the case records and represent the pressure of the patients before any medication was initiated. At the point of time when the study was begun the ocular pressure under topical antiglaucomatous therapy was determined. This was 20.0 ± 3.3 on the right and 19.9 ± 2.7 mmHg on the left. This deviation from the initial value is statistically highly significant.

After 2 weeks' application with metipranolol there was a further slight, but statistically highly significant reduction in the average inraocular pressure. It was now 18.6 ± 2.8 for the right and 18.6 ± 2.9 mmHg on the left eye. This average pressure value was maintained over the complete period of the study. The subsequent pressure values at the follow-up examinations after 8, 16 and 24 weeks after initiation of the study did not differ significantly from the initial value (2 weeks after metipranolol medication). The results are comparable with those obtained in the long-term study by Krieglstein [1], Dausch et al. [2], and Merté and Merkle [3], who all ascertained a lasting reduction in pressure under timolol eye drops, whereby Merté and Merkle [3] had to switch over more frequently from the weaker to the higher concentration. This was likewise the case in one of our patients. We could not detect any influence of treatment by metipranolol on the level of blood pressure or pulse frequency in any of our patients.

It must, nevertheless, be pointed out that patients with known asthma bronchiale or existing cardiac insufficiency were not included in the study.

As was expected there were not any changes in the width of pupils due to treatment with metipranolol nor could any influence on lacrimal secretion due to metipranolol be measured.

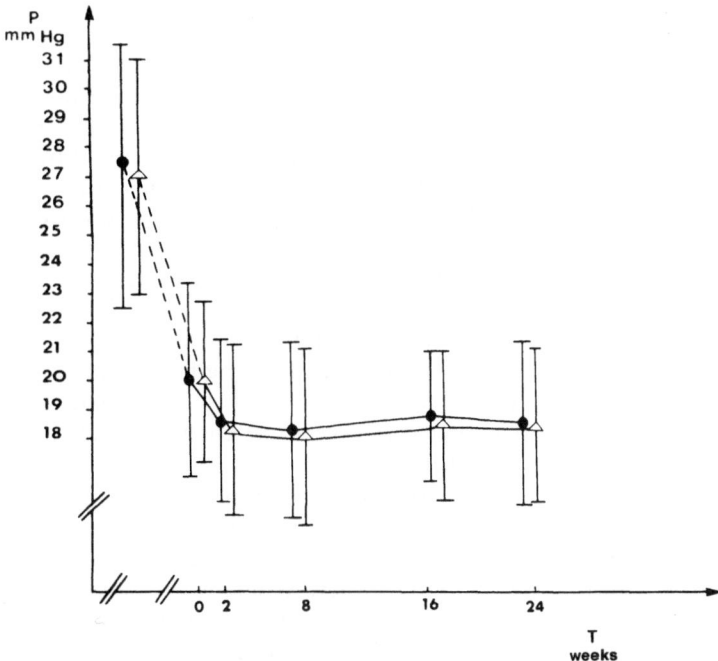

Fig. 1. Reaction of intraocular pressure in 47 patients under metipranolol treatment. ● right eye, △ left eye, $n = 47$. Mean values with standard deviation. The first value denotes pressure before any glaucoma therapy (so-called blank value). The second value was measured at the beginning of the study and represents the pressure obtained under previous glaucoma therapy but not under beta-blocking agents. The last four measured values represent the influence of metipranolol on ocular pressure

It must nevertheless be borne in mind that only the Schirmer's test I, which is known to measure the basic and irritative secretions simultaneously and in an unknown relationship to one another, was conducted. No doubt further studies, possibly including the Schirmer's test II, are necessary.

The average reduction in pressure due to metipranolol as against the blank value was about 30%. This value has likewise been mentioned in publications on other beta-blocking agents as such as timolol.

The objective tolerance was described as being good by the investigators. About 55% of all patients found the eye drops to be "neutral". The most frequent subjective side effect mentioned by the patients was an initial stinging upon instillation. This was reported by 45% of all patients. Only a few patients reported that this initial stinging abated during the course of the period of observation. Other subjective side effects such as itching, tearing, stabbing pain, headache or depression were mentioned by only 1—2 of the test persons and only at one point during the study. In consideration of the ubiquity of headache and occasional depression amongst older citizens and particularly in glaucoma patients, this figure seems to be remarkably low. Hypersensitivity reactions towards the product were observed in a total of 3 cases and ultimately resulted in 2 patients' discontinuing treatment with the drug. In another patient (female) the study had to be discontinued: this was because of asthma-like complaints which might possibly have been triggered off by metipranolol. Upon intensive questioning the patient reported that she had these complaints occasionally before the study began but she had not considered them serious enough to inform the investigator when stating her history.

In conclusion, it can be established that metipranolol is a beta-blocking agent which can be recommended in the form of eye drops for the treatment of glaucoma. During a period of 24 weeks metipranolol demonstrated a lasting effect, whereby the average reduction in pressure was about 30% as against the initial value. A loss in efficacy during the study period could not be observed. Metipranolol had no influence on pulse and blood pressure. The most frequent side effect complained of was a short initial stinging in the eyes after instillation but this did not result in treatment being discontinued at any time.

We wish to express our thanks to Prof. Dr. B. Schneider, Institute for Biometry at the Medizinische Hochschule Hannover for carrying out the statistical evaluation.

References

1. Krieglstein, G. K.: Die Wirkung von Timolol-Augentropfen auf den Augeninnendruck bei Glaucoma simplex. Klin. Mbl. Augenheilk. *172* 677 (1978).
2. Dausch, D., Michelson, W., Lorenz, E. D.: Die Langzeitbehandlung des Weitwinkelglaukoms mit Timolol. Klin. Mbl. Augenheilk. *174*, 127 (1979).

3. Merté, H.-J., Merkle. W.: Timolol-Augentropfen in der Glaukombehandlung. Ergebnisse einer Langzeitstudie. Klin. Mbl. Augenheilk.
177, 562 (1980).
4. Merté, H.-J., Mertz, M., Stryz, J.: Augendruck unter Metipranolol-
Einwirkung. In: Medikamentöse Glaukomtherapie (Krieglstein, G. K.,
Leydhecker, W., eds.). München: J. F. Bergmann. 1982.

Author's address: Priv.-Doz. Dr. H. von Denffer, Augenklinik und -poli-
klinik rechts der Isar der Technischen Universität München, Ismaninger
Strasse 22, D-8000 München 80, Federal Republic of Germany.

Results of a Long-term Study with Metipranolol

W. Kruse

Berlin

Since the introduction of pilocarpine in the treatment of glaucoma the topical application of beta-receptor blocking agents to the eye in order to reduce intraocular pressure has been the most radical change in glaucoma therapy. The various, for the patient often unpleasant disadvantages of treatment with miotics — loss of light due to contraction of pupils, myopisation and frequent instillation — no longer apply when beta-receptor blockers are used. During the last 3 months the beta-receptor blocker metipranolol (Betamann®) has been presented in 0.3% and 0.6% solutions as an effective alternative to timolol (Chibro-Timolol®), a beta-receptor blocker which has been widely used for some time. Today we wish to report on a long-term study which — after a pilot study had been conducted in the first 3 months of 1980 — was initiated in the second half of 1980 in our ophthalmological practice and is still being conducted.

This study relates only to glaucoma chronicum simplex. In each patient at least two of the three main criteria, which to a great extent allow a glaucoma to be diagnosed, were present:

elevated intraocular pressure above 24 mmHg,
scotomas which could not be explained otherwise
and
excavation of the optical nerve disk by at least half of its diameter and more.

In most cases the level of intraocular pressure was taken to be the mean value of a day curve.

10 patients participated in the pilot study in the first 3 months of 1980. 8 of these had been pretreated with miotic agents and 2 with Ophtorenin. From measurements taken at various times of

the day the study showed that within 14 days there was no vital change as against pretreatment when metipranolol, at that time in a 0.5% concentration, was used twice daily. In 2 patients with narrow chamber angles no other reaction of pressure was detected than in the remaining 8 patients with medium-wide to wide chamber angle.

In the second half of 1980 we began the long-term study which is still being conducted. The assessment of the first 6—12 months was part of a paper which has been published elsewhere. Today we shall report only on 25 patients who were included in the observation in our outpatient ophthalmological practice. 18 patients were female and 9 male. The mean age was 70.5 years, the youngest patient being 52 and the oldest 87 years of age.

By means of gonioscopy it was seen that 21 patients had medium-wide to wide chamber angles and 4 patients a narrow to sharp beak-shaped chamber angle which was barely just open.

All 25 patients had already been under treatment for glaucoma chronicum simplex at the beginning of the study. Pretreatment was as follows:

11 patients with carbachol,
9 patients with pilocarpine,
4 patients with aceclidin (Glaucotat®) and
1 patient with epiphrine.

In order to ensure as exact a judgement as possible when comparing results, all patients were instructed to instil regularly 1 drop of metipranolol into the eye at about 8 o'clock in the morning and 8 o'clock in the evening. The drops had to be kept inside the door of the refrigerator so that the patient himself could control the correct dosaging due to the feeling of coldness when instilling the drop. Both the time of the last treatment and the time of measuring pressure were registered. Drops were not instilled in the morning of the day that pressure was measured and the intraocular pressure was checked every 3—4 weeks. Within the scope of our controlling function it came to our notice again and again that some patients who were receiving other treatment for glaucoma were instilling the beta-receptor blocker timolol up to 4 times daily. Let it be mentioned here that 5 patients who instilled metipranolol 4 times daily instead of twice daily during 3 weeks did not show any further reduction in pressure than upon 2 instillations daily.

20 patients were given metipranolol 0.6% and the other 5 metipranolol 0.3%. Only those patients who maintained the therapy

throughout the complete period of observation were taken into consideration for the evaluation. Thus the following number of patients could be included when the results were being drawn up:

  6 months   25 patients,
  12 months   22 patients,
  18 months   15 patients,
  24 months   7 patients.

During the first 6 months none of the patients were excluded from the study but in the second period of observation 1 female patient had to undergo an operation because of a sudden deterioration in sight and visual field. Before the operation the intraocular pressure under treatment with metipranolol kept fluctuating between 18 and 25 mmHg, whereby the most common level was about 22 mmHg. Even at the beginning of pretreatment with miotica the visual acuity had already been distinctly reduced and the visual field very much limited. In another patient there was a sudden increase in pressure which could, however, be intercepted by the application of 2% pilocarpine along with metipranolol from the 16th month to the present. 1 female patient had to be changed over to another treatment because of a severe lid allergy to the vehicle in metipranolol drops.

In the third period of observation (12—18 months) 2 further female patients had to be excluded from the study because of allergy of the lids and conjunctiva to the vehicle in metipranolol eye drops. 1 patient had to undergo an operation because of a sudden increase in intraocular pressure over 30 mmHg. In this case additional treatment with pilocarpine, carbachol or Glaucotat anlong with metipranolol could only ward off the increase in pressure for a short ime. 1 patient did not come again to our practice and 3 others did not reach the 18-months limit.

In the last period of observation (18—24 months) a 4th patient had to discontinue treatment because of an allergy. 7 patients undergoing treatment with metipranolol have not yet reached the 24-months limit. From this it follows that the conclusions for the various periods of observation are based on numbers of patients decreasing at various rates.

4 out of 25 patients complained for a few days about a transient stinging after instillation. Most patients were surprised and pleased about the new light intensity they were experiencing again. On account of the absence of myopisation some patients had to have their glasses changed by up to 3 diopters tending towards hyperopia.

Our experience, however, shows that, after being switched over to treatment with beta-receptor blockers, patients should wait 2 months before new glasses are prescribed, provided that this does not involve difficulties at work.

With regard to objective changes, 4 patients, as mentioned above, manifested allergies of the lid and conjunctiva to the vehicle. After the allergic inflammations had disappeared, the pure vehicle solution without metipranolol was applied to these patients' eyes for a few days and after 4 days at the latest all 4 patients again showed the same inflammatory symptoms. In the first 6 months of treatment a further increase of an already present lens opacity with corresponding myopisation was seen in 1 patient but this did not progress in the following observation period of 18 months. After 19 months the same patient suffered from a central vein thrombosis in the left eye on account of a pronounced fundus hypertonicus et scleroticus.

As has been reported elsewhere in a paper dealing with metipranolol treatment in a multi-center long-term study, our 25 patients likewise exhibited a decrease in pressure of 33—34% with both metipranolol concentrations as against the blank value and a further reduction of 12% with metipranolol 0.3% and 22% with metipranolol 0.6% as against the intial value. We calculated the initial value to be the average value of the last 3—5 measurements of tension under pretreatment. With regard to the pressure reaction within these long-term studies over the complete observation period of 24 months hitherto, the results are based on the mean values of the 3 measurements taken at the given point of time in order to offset as far as possible individual fluctuations in terms of time.

This gave the following results:

	R	L
Beginning	19.3 / 19.4 mmHg	
6 months	20.3 / 19.6 mmHg	
12 months	19.6 / 19.9 mmHg	
18 months	19.9 / 20.1 mmHg	
24 months	19.3 / 18.6 mmHg	

The average fluctuations in pressure within the period of observation were not more than 1.0 mmHg for the right eye, 1.5 mmHg for the left eye or 2.5—2.7% of the mean pressure levels. It is known, however, that individually the results of single measurings deviate stronger from the mean pressure levels. It is noticeable that after 24 months of observation the intraocular pressure for the right eye corresponds to the tension at the beginning of the study and it is even somewhat lower for the left eye. Thus metipranolol maintains its initial pressure sinking effect over the complete period of observation of two years. In our patients the intraocular pressure was not seen to increase again after a good reduction in pressure at the beginning. The patients with narrow chamber angles showed no other conduct in pressure than those with medium-wide or wide chamber angles. 1 patient with a narrow iridocorneal angle exhibited the mentioned lid allergy, 2 have already been observed without complications for 24 months and 1 for 18 months.

The patients' blood pressure and pulse were checked frequently. No decrease was seen either in blood pressure values or pulse frequency.

Except for the female patient mentioned above all other patients did not exhibit any changes in visual functions or visual field.

Let me digress briefly from the subject. After the official introduction of metipranolol under the name Betamann® we have changed over 12 patients to this drug in the last few months. 7 patients had been pretreated with timolol, 1 patient with 1 drop of 2% pilocarpol eye oil in the evening and 1 patient with 2% pilocarpine 3 times daily and prostigmine eye ointment for the night. These 9 patients showed virtually the same conduct in pressure as before. 3 other patients who had previously instilled 2% pilocarpine eye drops 3 times daily and 2% pilocarpine eye oil for the night exhibited a further reduction in pressure of about 25—30%.

Again and again one of the last mentioned patients had at times to increase the dose of indometacine (Amuno®) because of rheumatic pains. A few days after increasing the dose, he constantly experienced pressure increases in the eye although the miotic therapy remained unchanged. After a subsequent decrease in the dose of indometacine, the intraocular pressure returned to normal. This pressure reaction to indometacine was observed frequently in our practice. However, it now became apparent that increases in pressure after the dose of indometacine had been increased could be intercepted by metipranolol. Long-term or frequent observations of this type have, however, still to be made.

After having been switched over from timolol to a corresponding concentration of metipranolol, 1 of these 12 patients complained about a transient stinging upon instilling the drops.

In conclusion, I should like to recapitulate the main results of the long-term study:

After the first observation period of 6 months 8 patients out of the initial number of 25 had to be excluded from the evaluation. 2 patients had to undergo an operation. 1 female patient received miotics in addition to metipranolol and a satisfactory reduction in pressure was obtained again. In 4 patients treatment was discontinued on account of an allergy of the lid and conjunctiva to the vehicle in metipranolol drops and 1 patient did not return as appointed to the controls after 12 months. From the subjective point of view tolerance was good. Most of the patients pretreated with miotics welcomed the advantages of treatment with metipranolol: instillation only twice daily and brighter sight.

Due to metipranolol the intraocular pressure was reduced satisfactorily in the 17 patients. During the period of observation of 2 years no loss could be ascertained in the pressure reducing effect and the tension did not increase again. Important side effects such as decreases in blood pressure or pulse beat were not observed. For the total of 37 patients the change from other glaucoma therapeutic agents to metipranolol prove to be unproblematic.

The statistical evaluation was carried out by Prof. Dr. phil. nat. B. Schneider, Department of Biometry in the Zentrum Biometrie, Medizinische Informatik und Medizintechnik der Medizinischen Hochschule Hannover.

Author's address: Dr. W. Kruse, Kaiserdamm 118, D-1000 Berlin 19.

Metipranolol Eye Drops — Clinical Suitability in the Treatment of Chronic Open Angle Glaucoma

D. Dausch, H. Brewitt, and R. Edelhoff

Eye Clinic, Medizinische Hochschule Hannover
(Director: Prof. Dr. H. Honegger),
Federal Republic of Germany

With 8 Figures

Introduction

Ever since Philips and associates [1] first reported in 1967 on an intraocular pressure sinking effect of the β-receptor blocking agent propranolol, more and more products of this group have been investigated as to their suitability for the treatment of glaucoma, whereby it became evident that, although many of these β-receptor blocking agents have an intraocular pressure sinking effect, they do in part differ considerably with regard to their action and side effects (Table 1).

The β-receptor blocking agent timolol-maleate (Chibro-Timoptol®) and bupranolol (Ophtorenin®) have been on the market in the Federal Republic of Germany for some years now and it has become impossible to imagine glaucoma therapy without them. The efficacy of these substances can be seen in that they are used with increasing success in the treatment of glaucoma and that, since the introduction of β-blocking agents, operations on a large number of glaucoma forms which are difficult to stabilize have either not been necessary or could at least be postponed.

Fortunately, in more recent times further substances have been developed from the range of β-blocking agents to enhance the choice of drugs for the treatment of glaucoma. One of these substances is metipranolol which we investigated with regard to its suitability to glaucoma therapy in the form of a clinical and animal experimental study.

Metipranolol hydrochloride (Betamann®, manufacturer: Dr. Mann Pharma, Berlin) was placed at our disposal as aqueous eye drop solutions in the concentrations 0.3 % and 0.6 %.

Table 1. *Survey of some β-receptor blocking agents which have so far been examined as to their suitability in glaucoma therapy*

	Intrinsic sympathomimetic activity (ISA)	Cardio-selective	Membrane-stabilizing	Reducing intraocular pressure
Propranolol	−	−	+	+
Sotalol	−	−	−	−
Practolol	+	+	−	+
Oxprenolol	+	−	+	+
Pindolol	+	−	−	+
Atenolol	−	+	−	+
Bupranolol	−	−	+	+
Timolol	−	−	(−)	+
Metoprolol	−	+	−	+
Metipranolol	−	−	(−)	+

This is a non-selective β-blocking agent without intrinsic sympathomimetic activity and with a minimum membrane-stabilizing effect [2—5]. Upon oral administration metipranolol is 4—8 times more effective than propranolol [6].

Methods

The initial pressure lowering effect of metipranolol was observed in a short-term study with 10 patients aged beween 50 and 90. This was a selected group of patients with chronic open angle glaucoma and, after a history of glaucoma of a few weeks up to 12 years, they were — with one exception — referred to us because they could no longer be regulated satisfactorily under previous treatment with miotics or adrenaline products.

The long-term effect was ascertained in altogether 41 patients aged between 42 and 83. 22 of these were newly diagnosed with a chronic open angle glaucoma or ocular hypertension, whereas the remaining 19 patients had already been pretreated.

23 out of 41 patients with significantly increased intraocular pressure values without treatment demonstrated neither scotomas nor glaucomatously changed papillae. Other 8 patients had discrete scotomas with normal papilla findings. 1 patient had a glaucomatous papilla without defective visual field. The remaining 9 patients had extensive scotomas with glaucomatously changed papillae.

1. Short-term Study

In order to obtain an insight into the initial pressure lowering effect of metipranolol eye drops, a 1-drop curve was prepared with 1 drop of 0.3 % metipranolol in 10 patients after discontinuing glaucoma therapy for at least 3—7 days. 1 drop of a placebo solution (BSS Ringer solution, Alcon) was administered to the other eye. By means of aplanation the intraocular pressure was measured 5 minutes before instillation and 5, 15, 30 minutes and 1, 2, 7, 12 and 24 hours after instillation.

Table 2. *Time schema for the long-term study with metipranolol*

	Before the beginning of the study	Therapy with metipranolol (weeks)			
		2	8	16	26
Intraocular pressure ..	x	x	x	x	x
Pupil width	x	x	x	x	x
Pulse and blood pressure	x	x	x	x	x
Visual field	x		x		x
Visual acuity	x	x			x
Refraction	x	x			x
Schirmer's test	x		x		x
Slit lamp	x	x	x	x	x
Ophthalmoscopy	x	x	x	x	x

On the second day of the trial the regular therapy of 2 times 1 drop metipranolol 0.3 % per eye was initiated. Tonographic examinations before beginning and on the 4th day of therapy were aimed at giving an indication of changes in outflow resistance or aqueous production under treatment with metipranolol.

2. Long-term Study

A long-term study was conducted over a period of 6 months. After any previous therapy had been discontinued for at least 3—7 days, treatment with 1 drop of metipranolol 0.3 % twice daily was initiated and, wherever necessary, the concentration was increased to 0.6 %.

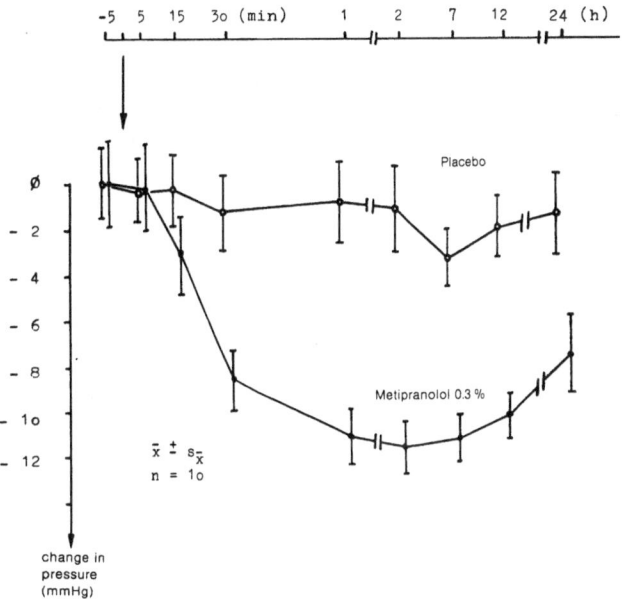

Fig. 1. Temporal course of intraocular pressure after single administration of 1 drop of metipranolol versus placebo

If the intraocular pressure could not be regulated under therapy with metipranolol alone, i. e. an additional drug or surgical intervention was necessary, the patients were excluded from further participation in the study.

Before treatment and during treatment with metipranolol control examinations were carried out according to an established time scheme (Table 2): as well as the measuring of intraocular pressure controls were carried out on the pupil width, visual field, sight and refraction. In order to rule out systemic side effects on the circulatory system, blood pressure and pulse frequency at rest were established.

In addition we carried out an experimental study in 3 rabbits (6 eyes) to rule out changes which might possibly occur on the cornea. For this metipranolol eye drops in a concentration of 0.6 % were applied twice daily to both eyes for 5 months. At the end of the experiment the animals were sacrificed and the corneae dissected for the transmission and scanning electron microscopic examinations.

Results

From the 1-drop curve (Fig. 1) it can be seen that the first reduction in pressure already set in 15 minutes after application of the drops. The greatest decrease in pressure can be registered in the time between 15 and 30 minutes.

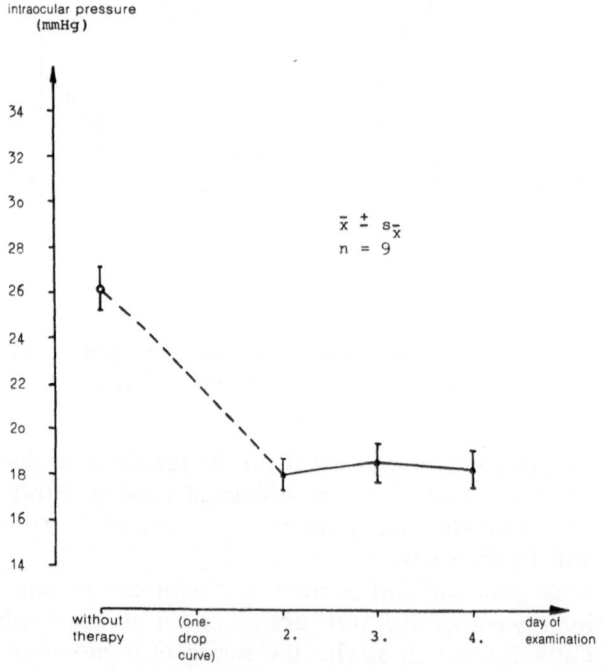

Fig. 2. Mean values of daily pressure curves on the last day before initiation of therapy and on the first 3 days under regular therapy of 1 drop metipranolol 0.3 % twice daily (2nd to 4th day of examination)

The lowest pressure value is reached after 2 hours and is on average 38 % below the initial value. After 24 hours the reduction in pressure is still 26 %.

In the 18 eyes of 9 patients in our short-term study a mean value of 26.16 ± 1.27 mmHg (Fig. 2) was found to be the average in the day pressure curve before therapy. On the 2nd day of examination a

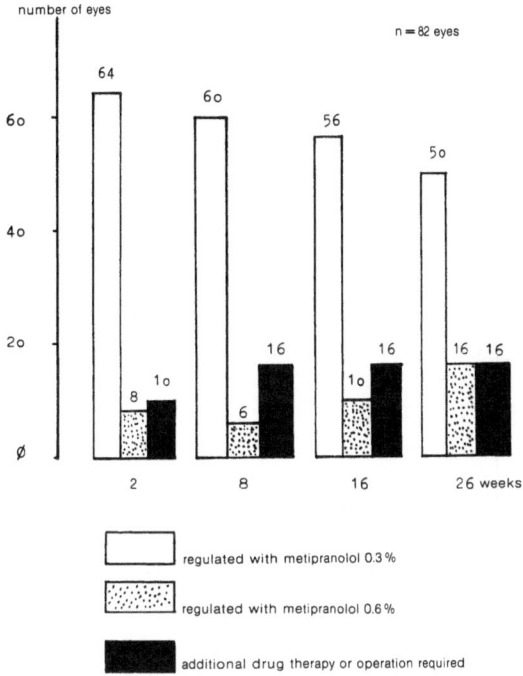

Fig. 3. Course of treatment under metipranolol 0.3 % and 0.6 % eye drops

significant decrease in pressure to an average of 18.05 ± 1.00 mmHg ($p < 0.001$) took place upon commencement of the regular therapy of 1 drop of metipranolol 0.3 % twice daily. The extent of the reduction in pressure decreased negligibly on the 3rd and 4th days of the examination.

The tonographic outflow facility c_{0-4} established at the same time in 16 glaucomatous eyes was on average 0.134 without therapy and 0.154 under therapy with metipranolol.

The difference is not significant statistically ($p > 0.05$). The same also applies to c_{L3-7}. The aqueous production assessed from the

values established tonographically decreases by an average of 20%
from an initial value of $2.23 \pm 0.31 \mu l/min$ to $1.79 \pm 0.33 \mu l/min$ —
taking the fact into consideration that tonography has but a limited
value in ascertaining aqueous production [7].

Out of the 82 glaucomatous eyes treated in our long-term study
64 eyes under metipranolol 0.3% and 8 eyes under metipranolol
0.6% could be adjusted within the first two weeks to an intraocular
pressure under 21 mmHg (Fig. 3).

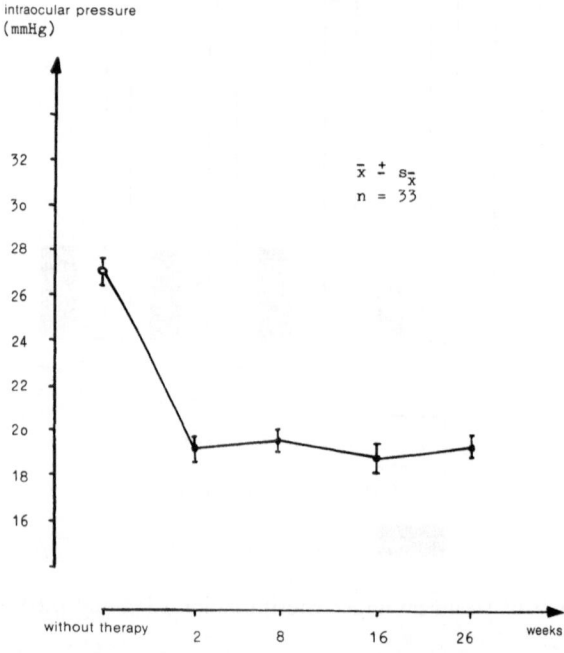

Fig. 4. The pressure reducing effect of metipranolol 0.3% and 0.6%
eye drops over a period of observation of half a year

In a further control after 8 weeks another 60 eyes could be regulated with metipranolol 0.3% and 6 eyes with metipranolol 0.6%.
The remaining 16 glaucomatous eyes could not be regulated
with metipranolol alone and thus they were excluded from our
study. In the further course of the study 10 eyes had to be switched
over from metipranolol 0.3% to a concentration of 0.6% because

the pressure values increased again. Thereafter pressure was like-wise regulated satisfactorily. This means that after half a year 80 % of the glaucomatous eyes treated were adjusted well.

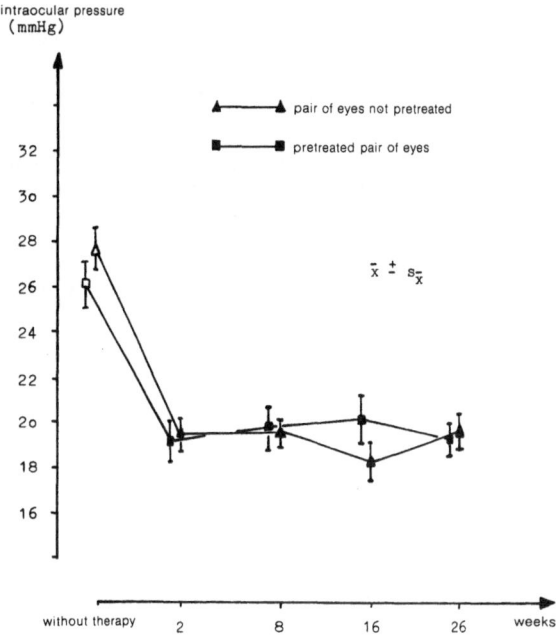

Fig. 5. Comparison of intraocular reducing effect of metipranolol 0.3 % and 0.6 % in non pretreated and pretreated glaucomatous eyes

The long-term effect of metipranolol eye drops was observed separately in 66 glaucomatous eyes (33 patients) which could be adjusted during the complete period of treatment with metipranolol (Fig. 4). The evaluation of the results shows that, under treatment with metipranolol 0.3 % or 0.6 % administered twice daily, the intraocular pressure could be reduced to a statistically significant extent from a mean initial value of 27.09 ± 0.63 mmHg to 19.30 ± 0.53 mmHg after two weeks ($p < 0.001$). This corresponds to a decrease in pressure of 29 %. This level could be maintained up to the end of the study with slight statistically non-significant fluctuations. After half a year the average intraocular pressure of the patients in the study was 19.50 ± 0.46 mmHg.

21 of the 33 patients in question were newly diagnosed cases for whom metipranolol treatment represented a first therapy. The remaining 12 patients had already been pretreated with other glaucoma drugs. A graphic illustration of these two groups of patients shows no vital differences in pressure reaction under metipranolol (Fig. 5).

The extent of the reduction in pressure under metipranolol also depends, as can be seen from the scattergram (Fig. 6), on the level of the initial intraocular pressure. At higher initial values the decreases in pressure were greater than at lower initial values, not only in terms of figures but also percentages: for example, with an untreated intraocular pressure of 23 mmHg ag was seen to have decreased by an average of about 5 mmHg or 22 % and an untreated eye with 33 mmHg decreased on average by 12 mmHg or 36 %.

The circulatory parameters (blood pressure and pulse) showed no statistically significant changes under metipranolol (Fig. 7) nor did the diameter of the pupil change under the drug. Visual acuity

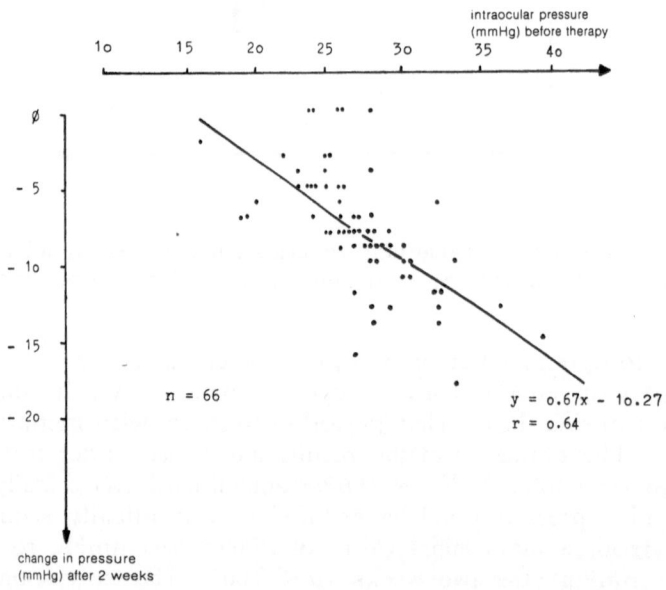

Fig. 6. Linear correlation between intraocular pressure before therapy and decrease in pressure after 2 weeks of regular treatment with 1 drop of metipranolol 0.3 % twice daily

remained unchanged in all patients. The determination of lacrimal production with the Schirmer's test likewise showed no significant influence due to the drug. Only in 2 patients was there a stronger reduction in lacrimal production and subjectively this was found to be annoying.

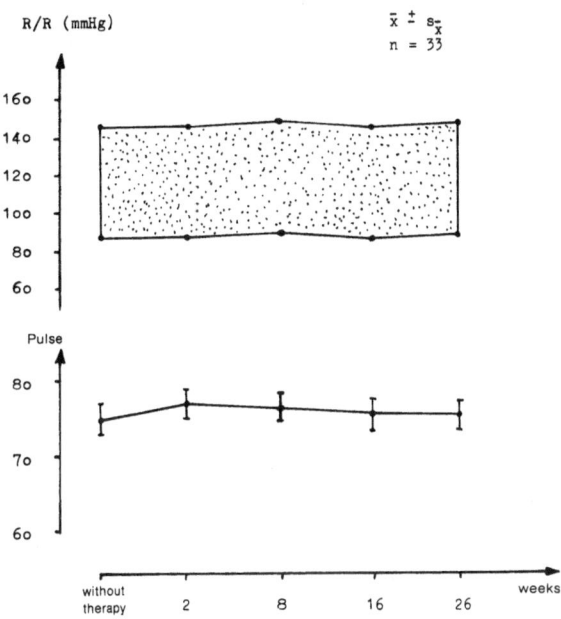

Fig. 7. Influence of metipranolol on blood pressure (above) and heart frequency (below)

As far as the subjective side effects of metipranolol are concerned, the most frequent complaint was stinging in the eye upon instillation and this disappeared again after few seconds. The complaints normally became fewer as treatment progressed (Table 3).

Objectively the eyes under therapy with metipranolol were examined biomicroscopically with the slit lamp and no pathological changes could be detected in the region of the anterior and medium segments. The perimetric determination demonstrated constant findings for the visual field in all patients throughout the duration of observation. The ophthalmoscopic examination likewise gave no indication of any progression of glaucomatous changes of the optic nerve.

The scanning electron microscopic findings depict light, medium-dark and dark epithelial cells. However, in comparison to the normal epithelium, the medium-dark and dark epithelial cells demonstrate a somewhat slighter microvilli covering on their surface. The reduced number of microappendices in the vicinity of the cell limit is evident (Fig. 8 a). Open cell limits cannot be detected.

Table 3. *Subjective side effects under topical treatment with metipranolol during a period of observation of 6 months*

$n = 33$	2 weeks			2 months			4 months			6 months		
	+	++	+++	+	++	+++	+	++	+++	+	++	+++
Itching	1		1	1						1		
Stinging	6	4	2	6	2	2	6	1	2	5	2	
Sensation of foreign body ...	2			4			2			2		
Photophobia ...												
Lacrimal flow ..	1	1	1	1	1		1	1		2		
Headache				1				1		1		
Tiredness	2			1			1			1		
Absent-mindedness												
Depressions												

+ slight   ++ medium   +++ severe

On studying the transmission electron microscopic pictures of the corneal preparations both the reduced and short microvilli covering (Fig. 8 b) and somewhat widened intracellular spaces on the surface cell layers become evident (Fig. 8 c). The rest of the histological structure seems to be unchanged.

Fig. 8. *a* Raster scanning electron microscopic picture of rabbit cornea: decreased number of microappendices in range of cell limit (arrows); SEM 5,000×. *b* Transmission electron microscopic picture of rabbit cornea: sparse microvilli (arrows) in intact outer plasma membrane; TEM 20,000×. *c* Transmission electron microscopic picture of rabbit cornea: extension of intercellular spaces (arrows); TEM 40 000×

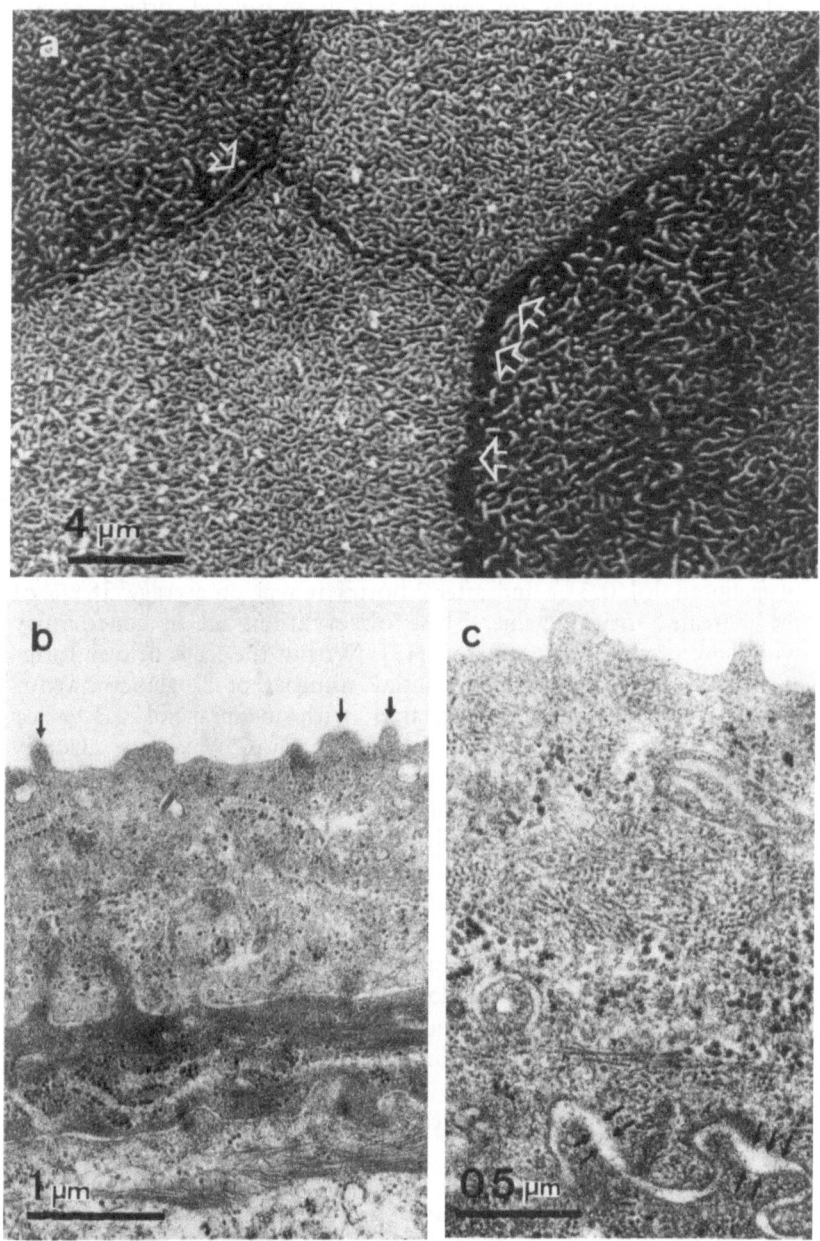

Fig. 8

The present findings are only detectable in isolated corneal areals and allow the conclusion that metipranolol — also after prolonged use — does not produce any serious side effects to the rabbit cornea.

Discussion

Metipranolol is a non-selective β-receptor blocking agent without intrinsic sympathomimetic activity and, compared to the propranolol, with a greater strength of action. The aqueous solution of metipranolol in the concentrations 0.3 % and 0.6 % was generally tolerated well on topical application to the eye. A sporadic incidence of irritation to the eye upon instillation is also known of timolol [8, 9, 10] and to a greater extent of propranolol [11] and metoprolol 12].

Our examinations showed that metipranolol eye drops are able to decrease elevated intraocular pressure in glaucomatous patients to a statistically significant and therapeutically satisfactory extent.

The intraocular pressure reducing action in 10 glaucomatous eyes already set in after 15 minutes following the application of 1 drop of metipranolol 0.3 % and after 2 hours it was on average 38 % of the untreated initial value. These observations are in conformity with those of other investigators [13]. Within the scope of our long-term study 66 eyes out of an initial number of 82 glaucomatous eyes, i. e. 80 %, could be regulated with metipranolol 0.3 % or 0.6 %. These are good results, similar to those which we already made in long-term studies with timolol eye drops [14].

When comparing the reduction in pressure obtained after 2 weeks with metipranolol with the individual initial pressure values before initiation of treatment, we noticed that patients with relatively high initial values mostly experienced a relatively high decrease in pressure. Evidently the extent of reduction in pressure depends on the level of the pressure before therapy. The same observation was also made in studies with timolol [15] and with bupranolol [16].

The mechanism of the intraocular pressure reducing action of β-receptor blocking agents including that of metipranolol has not been clarified. We did not find any statistically significant influence on the facility of outflow ascertained tonographically and thus came to similar results as are already known of timolol [17, 14] and bupranolol [16, 18]. After 1 month of therapy with pindolol, Bonomi and Steindler [19] found a slight increase in outflow facility but, according to their calculations, not more than a third of the pressure reducing effect can be attributed to this. The mechanism of action by which β-receptor blocking agents decrease intraocular pressure apparently ensues predominantly via a reduction in aqueous production [20, 21, 14]. The present study could also confirm this for metipranolol.

The circulatory parameters (blood pressure and pulse) measured at rest were not seen to be influenced by the drug. In this connection we should, however, like to remark that an examination of the circulatory parameters on physical exertion would also be important to be able to exclude any reduction of the physiological exercise tachycardia and the physiological increase in blood pressure which are dangerous to the eye already glaucomatously damaged.

In 31 out of 33 cases we found virtually no influence on lacrimal production. In 2 patients, however, the Schirmer's test provided decreased values. The development of dry eye can, therefore, not be exluded in isolated cases under therapy with metipranolol as has already been observed for timolol [22, 23]. Vigilance during topical β-blocker therapy to the eye, therefore, seems advisable, particularly if lacrimal production is already reduced.

Slit lamp findings gave no indication of objective changes in the region of the anterior and medium segment of the eye. This clinical observation showing good objective tolerance could be substantiated in animal experiments by means of scanning electron microscopic examinations on 6 rabbit corneae.

Altogether it can be ascertained that metipranolol provides us with a new active ingredient which is distinguished by its lasting pressure reducing effect and good subjective and objective tolerance. Longer clinical observation will prove whether and to what extent metipranolol offers advantages over the β-blockers, timolol and bupranolol, already in use.

The statistical evaluation was carried out by Prof. Dr. phil. nat. B. Schneider, Department of Biometry in the Zentrum Biometrie, Medizinische Informatik und Medizintechnik der Medizinischen Hochschule Hannover.

References

1. Phillips, C. I., Howitt, G., Rowlands, D. J.: Propranolol as ocular hypotensive agent. Br. J. Ophthalmol. 51, 222—226 (1967).
2. Simon, G., Dickhuth, H. H., Lindscheidt, U., Kindermann, W., Keul, J.: Hämodynamische und metabolische Auswirkungen der Beta-Rezeptorenblockade durch Metipranolol. Herz/Kreisl. 11, 134—140 (1979).
3. Scholtze, J., Smolarz, A.: Untersuchungen zur bronchospastischen Wirkung des β-Blockers Metipranolol bei Patienten mit chronischer Bronchitis. Therapiewoche 28, 876—882 (1978).

4. Bartsch, W., Dietmann, K., Leinert, H., Sponer, G.: Cardiac action of Carazolol and Methypranol in comparison with other β-receptor blockers. Arzneim. Forsch./Drug Res. 27 (I), 1022—1026 (1977).

5. Bartsch, W., Sponer, G., Dietmann, K.: Experiments in animals on the pharmacological effects of Metipranolol in comparison with Propranolol and Pindolol. Arzneim. Forsch./Drug. Res. 27 (II), 2319—2322 (1977).

6. Dietmann, K., Döring, G., Akpan, W., Schröter, E.: Die Bestimmung vergleichbarer beta-sympathikolytischer Dosen von Methypranol und Propranolol anhand der Herzfrequenz in Ruhe und unter submaximaler Belastung bei gesunden Probanden. Herz/Kreisl. 9, 783—789 (1977).

7. Leydhecker, W.: Manual der Tonographie für die Praxis. Berlin — Heidelberg — New York: Springer. 1977.

8. Nielsen, N. V.: Timolol — Hypotensive effect, used alone and in combination for treatment of increased intraocular pressure. Acta Ophthalmol. 56, 504—509 (1978).

9. McMahon, Ch. D., Shaffer, R. N., Hoskins, H. D., Hetherington, J.: Adverse effects experienced by patients taking Timolol. Am. J. Ophthalmol. 88, 736—738 (1979).

10. Wilson, R. P., Spaeth, G. L., Poryzees, E.: The place of Timolol in the practice of ophthalmology. Ophthalmology 87, 451—454 (1980).

11. Vale, J., Gibbs, A. C. C., Phillips, C. I.: Topical Propranolol and ocular tension in the human. Br. J. Ophthalmol. 56, 770—775 (1972).

12. Bucheli, J., Aeschlimann, J., Gloor, B.: Die Wirkung von Metoprolol-Augentropfen auf den Augeninnendruck. Klin. Mbl. Augenheilk. 177, 146—150 (1980).

13. Dienstbier, E., Růžičková, E., Čepelík, J.: Metipranolol v léčbe glaucomu. Čs. Oftal. 37, 5—12 (1981).

14. Dausch, D., Michelson, W., Lorenz, E. D.: Die Langzeitbehandlung des Weitwinkelglaukoms mit Timolol. Klin. Mbl. Augenkeilk. 174, 127—135 (1979).

15. Nielsen, N. V., Eriksen, J. S.: Timolol in maintenance treatment of ocular hypertension and glaucoma. Acta Ophthalmol. 57, 1070—1077 (1979).

16. Krieglstein, G. K., Sold-Darseff, J., Leydhecker, W.: The intraocular pressure response of glaucomatous eyes to topically applied Bupranolol. Graefes Arch. Klin. Exp. Ophthalmol. 202, 81—86 (1977).

17. Zimmermann, Th. J., Harbin, R., Pett, M., Kaufman, H. E.: Timolol and facility of outflow. Invest. Ophthalmol. Visual Sci. 16, 623—624 (1977).

18. Stiegler, G.: Bupranolol-Augentropfen (Ophtorenin®) in der Glaukom-Dauertherapie. Klin. Mbl. Augenheilk. 174, 267—275 (1979).

19. Bonomi, L., Steindler, P.: Effect of pindolol on intraocular pressure. Br. J. Ophthalmol. 59, 301—303 (1975).

20. Coakes, R. L., Brubaker, R. F.: The Mechanism of Timolol in lowering intraocular pressure in the normal eye. Arch. Ophthalmol. *96,* 2045—2048 (1978).

21. Yablonski, M. E., Zimmerman, Th. J., Waltman, S. R., Becker, B.: A fluorophotometric study of the effect of topical timolol on aqueous humor dynamics. Exp. Eye Res. *27,* 135—142 (1978).

22. Bonomi, L., Zavarise, G., Noya, E., Michieletto, St.: Effects of Timolol Maleate on tear flow in human eyes. Graefes Arch. Klin. Exp. Ophthalmol. *213,* 19—22 (1980).

23. Nielsen, N. V., Eriksen, J. S.: Timolol — Transitory manifestations of dry eyes in long term treatment. Acta Ophthalmol. *57,* 418—424 (1979).

Authors' address: Prof. Dr. D. Dausch, Augenklinik, Medizinische Hochschule Hannover, Karl-Wiechert-Allee 9, D-3000 Hannover 61, Federal Republic of Germany.

Prophylaxis of an Iatrogenic Increase in Intraocular Pressure

P. Schmitz-Valckenberg

Ophthalmological Department, Hospital Evangelisches Stift, Koblenz
(Executive doctors: Dr. D. F. Brambring and Dr. P. Schmitz-Valckenberg),
Federal Republic of Germany

Sudden increases in intraocular pressure are often caused by drug treatment or surgery. The local or systemic application of atropine-like drugs can elevate intraocular pressure by the increase in flow resistance or due to an iris blockade becoming manifest.

Drugs with atropine-like effects include anti-Parkinson agents, antihistaminics, spasmolytics, derivatives for the dilatation of the coronary vessels, psychotropic drugs including tricyclic antidepressives and phenothiazines, corticosteroids and sympathomimetics.

In particular, hypertension occurring intraoperatively can be attributed to a haemorrhage.

Furthermore, transient increases in intraocular pressure are well-known symptoms during the first days following cataract extractions. These are frequently observed when alpha-chymotrypsin is used for zonulolysis but they can also occur when this ferment is not used.

In a study on 20 cataract operations without enzyme an increase in intraocular pressure of 26—50 mmHg (average 29 mmHg) was ascertained in the first 48 hours following the operation. The highest increase was observed in these patients at 6.8 hours after surgery [7].

In the following we shall report on the results of a randomised double-blind study with metipranolol eye drops to prevent elevation of intraocular pressure after cataract extraction.

Methods

40 eyes of 40 patients, who were admitted to the hospital for a routine cataract extraction, are involved in the study. The age, sex and period of observation are given in Table 1. Only patients known by the doctor to have senile cataracts were included in the study. Indications excluding patients from the study were alle forms of glaucoma, opticus processes, inflammatory eye diseases and intraoperative complications. On account of the possible systemic side effects of metipranolol, patients with severe angiocardiopathy and obstructive airways diseases were likewise excluded from participating.

Table 1

	Treated with metipranolol	Treated with placebo
Number of eyes	20	20
Mean age of patients	75 years	72 years
Men/women	9/11	8/12
Period of observation	10 days altogether	

At 7 p. m. on the evening before the operation 1 drop of metipranolol 0.6% or a placebo preparation was administered to the eyes to be operated and then in each phase at 7 a. m. and 7 p. m. on the following 5 days. By means of applanation the intraocular pressure was measured on the evening before the operation and in each case at 8 a. m. and 5 p. m. on the following days. In addition, a preparation containing an antibiotic was administered postoperatively 3 times daily during this period.

All patients received a retrobulbar injection of 4—5 ml of a topical anaesthetic. After the corneoscleral opening, using the 2-stage method of incision, application of a peripheral iridectomy and injection of 1 cm^3 alpha-chymotrypsin the lens was extracted intracapsularly and without loss of corpus with the cryo-stiletto. The wound was closed with an uninterrupted Tübingen suture (10/0 silk). Two operating surgeons participated in this study.

Results

The results of the measurements of intraocular pressure is given in Table 2 for all 40 patients.

Table 2

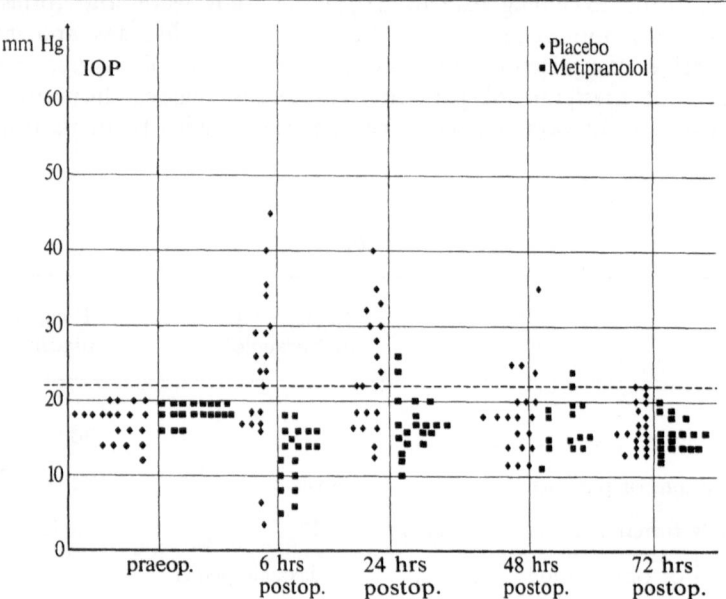

13 out of 20 untreated patients exhibited an increase in intra-ocular pressure within the first 24 hours, whereas only 2 of the patients treated with metipranolol experienced an elevation of ocular pressure during this time.

The highest increases in intraocular pressure were found at the first measurement 6 hours after the operation. 9 eyes treated with metipranolol showed a distinctly reduced ocular pressure under 15 mmHg 6 hours after the operation (t test, $p < 0.05$). 24 hours after the operation the intraocular pressure of 15 eyes treated with metipranolol had reached normal values (between 15 and 20 mmHg).

On the second day after the operation, elevated values were ascertained in only 4 of the eyes treated with the placebo and 2 with metipranolol. On the third day after the operation, all 40 eyes had reached normal values. We intentionally dispensed with information on other results (particularly with regard to sight) as our patients were observed consistently for only 7 days. In none of the

40 patients did we observe postoperatively any hyphaemia, end-ophthalmitis, wound rupture, flat anterior chamber, pupillary block, retinal detachment or any more pronounced corneal edema. None of the patients showed clinical signs of a systemic side effect after metipranolol eye drops.

Discussion

The results of this study confirm the frequent occurrence of elevated intraocular pressure after cataract extractions involving the use of alpha-chymotrypsin. 60% of our patients (12 out of 20) showed an increase in pressure between 22 and 40 mmHg in the first 24 hours after the operation.

Moreover, we ascertained in our test series that the highest increases in pressure occur within the first 24 hours after the operation. In all cataract extractions following a normal course normal pressure values are obtained again in the following days. We could not find any reason for this transient increase in intraocular pressure. However, for this study we intentionally selected only such patients as — under the same initial conditions from the doctor's point of view — exhibited an uncomplicated operation and a normal postoperative course.

Particular value was placed on the non-occurrence of bleeding in the anterior chamber during or after the operation. Blood occurring intraoperatively was immediately washed out of the anterior chamber. This seemed to us important, as there might be a relationship between intraocular pressure and the occurrence of blood in the anterior chamber [2, 5, 8]. Furthermore, no frequent occurrence of bleeding was observed when metipranolol was used.

Our results distinctly show a significant reduction in ocular pressure after the application of metipranolol within the first few hours after cataract extraction. Only in 2 patients treated with metipranolol did we see an increase in pressure between 24 and 26 mmHg during the first 24 hours.

These findings conform with those of other investigators using timolol or acetazolamide [6, 8, 10, 11]. These drugs are suitable for the prevention of elevated intraocular pressure in the first 24 hours.

In comparison with timolol we were able to find values under 15 mmHg in 13 eyes treated with metipranolol at the measurement taken 6 hours after the operation. Haiman and Phelps [10] report on pressure values significantly above 15 mmHg in 12 eyes treated with timolol during the same time.

As in the further course of the postoperative phase the ocular pressure values are similar in the treated and untreated eyes, a prophylactic treatment with beta-receptor blocking agents does not seem advisable after the third day following the operation. Hayreh [9] reported on 11 patients who developed an opticus neuropathy in the anterior segment immediately after the cataract extraction. As a significantly increased ocular pressure was ascertained in the majority of these patients during the first few days after the operation, the author considers this to be the main cause for the development of opticus neuropathy.

In conclusion the following can be established from reports in literature and on the basis of our own results:

1. In cataract extractions following a normal course increases in intraocular pressure occur in the first 24 hours after the operation in the majority of cases.

2. Metipranolol as a beta-receptor blocking agent is particularly suitable for lowering intraocular pressure effectively in this postoperative phase.

3. Upon the routine application of beta-receptor blocking agents complications do not occur either before or after the operation.

4. It seems recommendable to use beta-receptor blocking agents before operations and immediately after operations on patients with extended arteriosclerotic changes in order to present effectively any anterior opticus neuropathy [9].

References

1. Giardini, A., Paliaga, G. P.: Comportamento del tono dopo estrazione di cataratta. Ann. Ottalmol. Clin. Oculist 88, 551—563 (1962).

2. Giardini, A., Paliaga, G. P.: Cataract extraction with optimum wound closure. Br. J. Ophthalmol. 84, 133—138 (1964).

3. Kirsch, R. E.: Glaucoma following cataract extraction associated with use of alpha-chymotrypsin. Arch. Ophthalmol. 72, 612—620 (1964).

4. Galin, M. A., Barasch, K. R., Harris, L. S.: Enzymatic zonulysis and intraocular pressure. Am. J. Ophthalmol. 61, 690—696 (1966).

5. Pape, R.: Vergleichende Messungen zu Schnitt- und Nahtverfahren bei der Katarakt-Extraktion. Graefes Arch. Klin. Exp. Ophthalmol. 173, 199—216 (1967).

6. Rich, W. J. C. C.: Further studies on early post-operative ocular hypertension following cataract extraction. Trans. Ophthalmol. Soc. U. K. 89, 639—645 (1969).

7. Rich, W. J., Radtke, N. D., Cohan, B. E.: Early ocular hypertension after cataract extraction. Br. J. Ophthalmol. *58*, 725—731 (1974).

8. Galin, M. A., Lin, L. L. K., Obstbaum, S. A.: Cataract extraction and intraocular pressure. Trans. Ophthalmol. Soc. U. K. *98*, 124—127 (1978).

9. Hayreh, S. S.: Anterior ischemic optic neuropathy. IV. Occurrence after cataract extraction. Arch. Ophthalmol. *98*, 1410—1416 (1980).

10. Haimann, M. H., Phelps, Ch. D.: Prophylactic timolol for the prevention of high intraocular pressure after cataract-extraction. Am. Acad. Ophthalmol. *88*, 233—238 (1981).

11. Packer, A. J., Fraioli, A. J., Epstein, D. L.: The effect of timolol and aztetazolamide on transient intraocular pressure elevation following cataract extraction with alpha-chymotrypsin. Am. Acad. Ophthalmol. *88*, 239—243 (1981).

Author's address: Dr. P. Schmitz-Valckenberg, Augenabteilung, Krankenhaus Evangelisches Stift, Johannes-Müller-Strasse 7, D-5400 Koblenz, Federal Republic of Germany.

Regulating Pressure in Various Forms of Glaucoma with Metipranolol Eye Drops

N. Demmler

Passau

With 7 Figures

In the last few years some beta-receptor blocking agents have been introduced with varying success to ophthalmology (Demmler, N., 1980 [2]). Of these I wish to mention bupranolol (Demmler, N., 1980 [3, 4]; Krieglstein, G. K., and associates, 1979 [10]; Stiegler, G., 1979 [14]; Oancea, I., 1979 [12]; Leydhecker, W., Krieglstein, G. K., 1979 [11]) and timolol (Dausch, D., and associates, 1979 [1]; Merté, H. J., Merkle, W., 1980 [17, 18]; Demmler, N., Müller-Bardorff, G., 1980 [7]; Demmler, N., 1982 [8]; Katz, I. M., 1979 [9]) which have been successfully used in numerous patients. Other beta-receptor blocking agents such as propranolol (Phillips, C. I., and associates, 1967 [13]) have not come up to expectations.

This paper shall now study the extent to which the beta-receptor blocking agent metipranolol (Betamann®) is commendable for the therapy of various forms of glaucoma. So far but a few papers are available on metipranolol: Merté, H.-J., and associates, 1982 [15], and Draeger, J., and associates, 1982 [16].

Methods

All patients had glaucoma in both eyes. The age of the patients was between 50 and 82 years. All patients had already been pre-treated with various miotics. There was either a decompensation under this therapy or the previous therapy could not be continued because of subjective complaints. Blood pressure controls were carried out regularly — at least once a month — in all patients and, furthermore, controls of vision and visual field (Goldmann perimeter) were carried out. The intraocular pressure was measured regularly by means of applanation and also in the form of daily pressure measurements.

Furthermore, the patients were constantly examined with the slit lamp, ophthalmoscope and gonioscope.

Results

Effect of Metipranolol in Glaucoma Chronicum Simplex (Open Angle Glaucoma)

5 patients (3 men, 2 women) with open angle glaucoma received metipranolol eye drops 0.3 % topically twice daily. The patients were controlled regularly for a year. The mean pressure values before treatment were 31 mmHg without therapy. Under treatment with metipranolol there was a reduction in intraocular pressure to values between 24 and 22 mmHg. The mean reduction in pressure is about 8 mmHg (Fig. 1). All patients tolerated the drug well and visus and visual field remained unchanged.

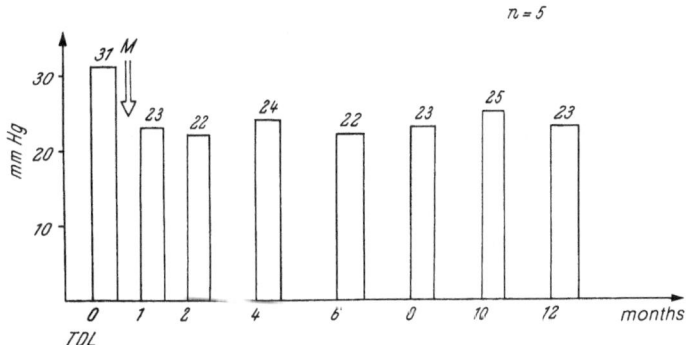

Fig. 1. Metipranolol in glaucoma chronicum simplex (open angle glaucoma — mean values from daily pressure measurements). *M* metipranolol, *TDL* daily pressure without drug, *n* number of cases

A second group of patients with open angle glaucoma were given metipranolol eye drops 0.3 % along with a miotic (3 times 1 % pilocarpine eye drops, 2 times 1.5 % isopto-carbachol eye drops). Under this combination therapy the mean pressure values can be reduced significantly. The starting value is 28 mmHg and the control values between 24 and 21 mmHg (Fig. 2). No change can be ascertained in blood pressure values. Vision and visual field remain unchanged. Subjective complaints are not registered.

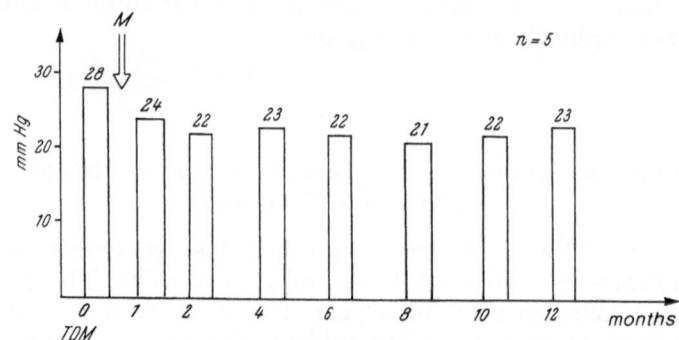

Fig. 2. Effect of metipranolol in combination with miotics in glaucoma chronicum simplex (open angle glaucoma — mean values from daily pressure measurements). *M* metipranolol, *TDM* daily pressure with miotics, *n* number of cases

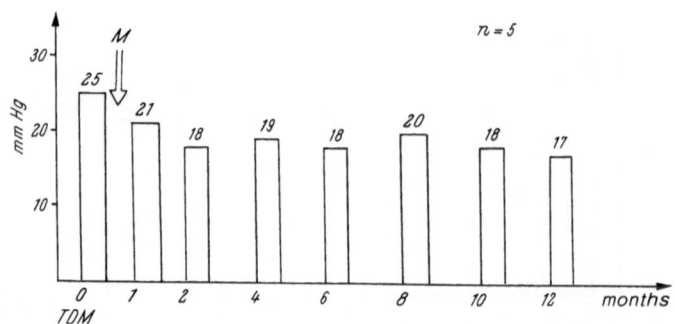

Fig. 3. Effect of metipranolol in combination with a miotic in glaucoma chronicum congestivum (narrow angle glaucoma — mean values from daily pressure measurements). *M* metipranolol, *TDM* daily pressure with miotics, *n* number of cases

Glaucoma Chronicum Congestivum

A further group of patients with narrow angle glaucomas received metipranolol along with a miotic (Fig. 3). The miotic therapy applied was pilocarpine eye drops 2% in two cases, isopto-carbachol eye drops 1.5% in two cases and glaucostat eye drops in one case.

By means of combination therapy the intraocular pressure could be reduced by about 5 mmHg. The initial values were at 25 mmHg, and after the application of metipranolol values between 21 and 18 mmHg were measured over the complete period of one year. Vision and visual field were unchanged. The blood pressure remained constant under therapy with metipranolol. Subjective complaints were not stated.

Glaucoma in Aphakic Eyes

A group of patients with glaucoma in aphakic eyes (3 patients) could be adjusted satisfactorily under therapy with metipranolol eye drops 0.3 % alone. The initial values before therapy were 26 mmHg.

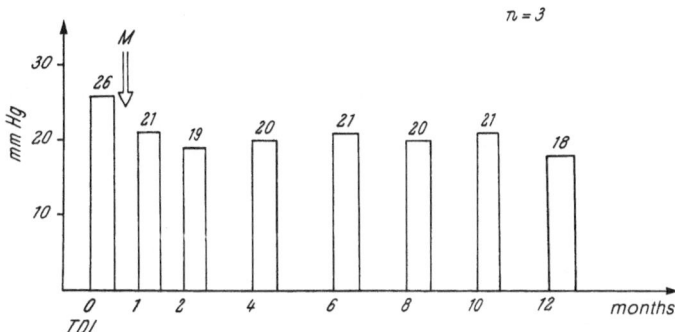

Fig. 4. Metipranolol effect on glaucoma in aphakic eye (mean values from daily pressure measurements). M metipranolol, TDL daily pressure without drug, n number of cases

Under therapy, pressure values between 18 and 21 mmHg were measured (Fig. 4). Vision and visual field remained constant. The blood pressure did not show any particular fluctuations.

In another group of patients (3 patients), likewise with glaucomas in aphakic eyes, a combination therapy of a miotic (3 times 1% pilocarpine eye drops) and 0.3% metipranolol eye drops could be carried out for a year. The initial values with pilocarpine but without metipranolol were 29 mmHg. Under the combination therapy a significant reduction in pressure to values of 22 mmHg could be ascertained (Fig. 5). The vision and visual field remained unchanged: the blood pressure did not decrease.

Exfoliative Glaucoma

3 patients with exfoliative glaucomas exhibited a significant reduction in pressure under treatment with metipranolol. The initial

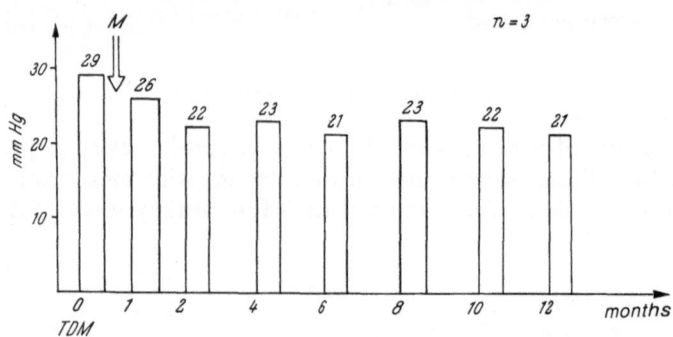

Fig. 5. Effect of metipranolol in combination with miotics on glaucoma
in aphakic eye (mean values from daily pressure measurements). M metipranolol, TDM daily pressure with miotic, n number of cases

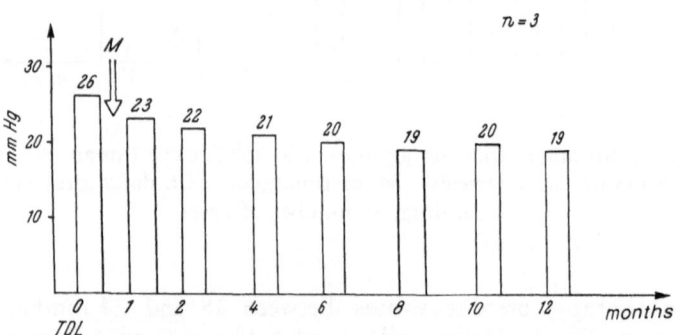

Fig. 6. Effect of metipranolol on exfoliative glaucoma (mean values from
daily pressure measurements). M metipranolol, TDL daily pressure without drug, n number of cases

value was 26 mmHg. Under metipranolol therapy values between
19 and 23 mmHg were ascertained (Fig. 6). The vision and visual
field remained unchanged. The blood pressure was constant. Subjective complaints were not registered.

Neovascular Glaucoma

Another group of patients which had already been treated with a miotic (0.5 % pilocarpine eye drops) on account of neovascular glaucomas did not show any satisfactory adjustment in pressure under therapy with pilocarpine alone. The mean values were about 32 mmHg. Due to the additional treatment with metipranolol eye drops 0.3 % we did succeed in reducing the mean ocular pressure

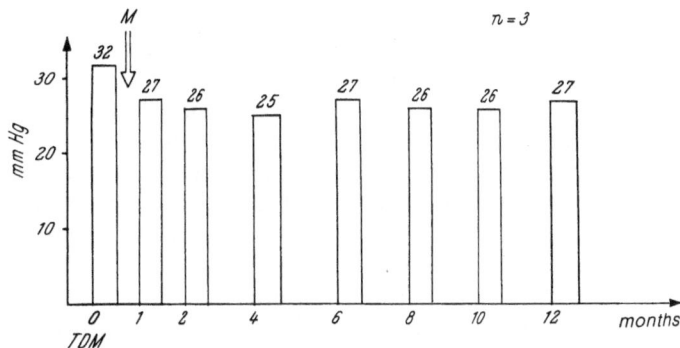

Fig. 7. Effect of metipranolol in combination with miotics on neovascular glaucomas (mean values from daily pressure measurements). M metipranolol, TDM daily pressure with drug, n number of cases

by about 5 mmHg. The values under the combination therapy were between 27 and 25 mmHg (Fig. 7). Subjective complaints were not registered.

Discussion

All patients had clearly better pressure values with metipranolol than with the usual miotics, i. e. a good regulation in pressure could be obtained under treatment with metipranolol alone. The blood pressure values remained unchanged nor was any deterioration in the finding for the visual field ascertained after 12 months of therapy with metipranolol. The vision likewise remained unchanged. Any different reduction in pressure was not detectable in the various forms of glaucoma such as angle glaucoma, narrow angle glaucoma, glaucoma associated with aphakia, exfoliative glaucoma and neovascular glaucoma. Any decrease in the drug-induced reduction in pressure was likewise not detected during treatment lasting one year.

Subjective complaints were not mentioned by the patients. Never-theless, metipranolol like other beta-receptor blocking agents, e. g. timolol or bupranolol, should not be administered to patients with asthma bronchiale (Demmler, N., Müller-Bardorff, G., 1980 [5]; Demmler, N., 1980 [6]).

Treatment with metipranolol eye drops alone is not indicated in narrow angle glaucoma, as an acute closing of the iridocorneal angle could occur under this treatment. Because of this, metipran-olol should be administered in combination with a miotic in cases of narrow angle glaucoma.

With regard to open angle glaucoma the pressure in one group of patients was regulated well under treatment with metipranolol alone (Fig. 1), whereas in a second group of patients with open angle glaucoma a satisfactory regulation in pressure could only be obtained with a combination therapy of a miotic and metipranolol (Fig. 2). A reason for this might well be the varying intensity of the individual glaucomas. In principle treatment with metipranolol alone does seem possible in open angle glaucoma as there is no risk of a closure of the iridocorneal angle.

Also in the group of patients with glaucoma associated with apha-kia, pressure is regulated well either with metipranolol alone (Fig. 4) or with a combination therapy of a miotic and metipranolol (Fig. 5).

In the group with exfoliative glaucomas significant reductions in pressure are exhibited under treatment with metipranolol (Fig. 6). Even in the case of neovascular glaucoma which is difficult to regu-late metipranolol produces an improvement in pressure reduction as compared to therapy with miotics alone, although the reduction in pressure in this group does not come within the range of normal (Fig. 7).

A great advantage of therapy with metipranolol is that hitherto decompensated forms of glaucoma which made an operation abso-lutely essential can now be stabilized, particularly due to combina-tion therapy of a miotic with metipranolol, so that an operation can be avoided. The stability of visual field findings over a period of a year seem to confirm that under treatment with metipranolol a satisfactory blood circulation is available in the capillary range of the nervus opticus. However, further controls are recommended.

References

1. Dausch, D., Michelson, W., Lorenz, E. D.: Die Langzeitbehandlung des Weitwinkelglaukoms mit Timolol. Klin. Mbl. Augenheilk. *174*, 127 (1979).

2. Demmler, N.: Beta-Rezeptorenblocker in der Ophthalmologie. Med. Mo. Pharm. *3*, 174—179 (1980).

3. Demmler, N.: Langzeitbehandlung des Weitwinkelglaukoms mit Bupranolol. Klin. Mbl. Augenheilk. *177*, 523—526 (1980).

4. Demmler, N.: Glaukomtherapie mit Bupranolol über ein Jahr. Zschr. für Prakt. Augenheilk. *4*, 27—29 (1980).

5. Demmler, N., Müller-Bardorff, G.: Timolol-Langzeitbehandlung des Weitwinkelglaukoms in der Praxis. Klin. Mbl. Augenheilk. *177*, 91—93 (1980).

6. Demmler, N.: Langzeitbehandlung bei Engwinkelglaukom mit Bupranolol-Augentropfen. Klin. Mbl. Augenheilk. *177*, 618—621 (1980).

7. Demmler, N., Müller-Bardorff, G.: Timolol — therapeutische Möglichkeiten in der Praxis bei Engwinkelglaukom (Langzeitbehandlung). Klin. Mbl. Augenheilk. *177*, 94—96 (1980).

8. Demmler, N.: Grenzen der Timololbehandlung. Folia ophthal. (Leipzig) *7*, 53—56 (1982).

9. Katz, I. M.: Wirksamkeit und Sicherheit der Langzeitbehandlung mit Timolol-Augentropfen beim chronischen Offenwinkelglaukom. Klin. Mbl. Augenheilk. *175*, 225 (1979).

10. Krieglstein, G. K., Sold-Darseff, J., Leydhecker, W.: The Intraocular pressure response of glaucomatous eyes to topically applied Bupranolol. Graefes Arch. klin. Ophthalmol. *202*, 81—86 (1977).

11. Leydhecker, W., Krieglstein, G. K.: The intraocular pressure responses of Pranolol (Ophtorenin) and Methazolamide (Neptazane) in glaucomatous eyes. Graefes Arch. klin. Ophthalmol. *210*, 135—140 (1979).

12. Oancea, I., Trif, V.: Über die Drucksenkung mit Bupranolol in wäßriger Lösung beim chronischen Glaukom simplex. Klin. Mbl. Augenheilk. *174*, 739—744 (1979).

13. Phillips, C. I., Howitt, G., Rowlands, D. J.: Propranolol as ocular hypotensive agent. Brit. J. Ophthalmol. *51*, 222—226 (1967).

14. Stiegler, G.: Bupranolol-Augentropfen (Ophtorenin) in der Glaukom-Dauertherapie. Klin. Mbl. Augenheilk. *174*, 267—275 (1979).

15. Merté, H. J., Mertz, M., Stryz, J., München: Augendruck unter Metipranolol-Einwirkung. In: Medikamentöse Glaukomtherapie (Krieglstein, G. K., Leydhecker, W., eds.), pp. 189—193. München: Bergmann. 1982.

16. Draeger, J., Buhr-Unger, H., Winter, R., Hamburg: Die Wirkung von Beta-Rezeptoren-Blockern auf die Hornhautsensibilität. In: Medikamentöse Glaukomtherapie (Krieglstein, G. K., Leydhecker, W., eds.), pp. 195—199. München: Bergmann. 1982.

17. Merté, H.-J., Merkle, W.: Ergebnisse einer Doppelblindstudie mit verschiedenen Konzentrationen von Pilocarpin und Timolol zur Glaukombehandlung. Klin. Mbl. Augenheilk. *177*, 443—450 (1980 a).

18. Merté, H.-J., Merkle, W.: Timolol-Augentropfen in der Glaukombehandlung. Ergebnisse einer Langzeitstudie. Klin. Mbl. Augenheilk.
177, 562—571 (1980 b).

Author's address: Dr. N. Demmler, Augenarzt, Ludwigsstrasse 2,
D-8390 Passau, Federal Republic of Germany.

Supplementary Comments
from the Discussion at the Metipranolol Symposium

Compiled and reviewed by

J. Stryz and H. v. Denffer

The following is a brief summary of some of the topics of discussion on the main issue of the symposium. These seem relevant to the authors of the report and are included in this book. As some of the numerous comments during the discussion partly covered the same ground, it seemed commendable to group these into sections dealing with the main points of interest.

Topical Subjective Tolerance of Beta-blocking Agents in General and of Metipranolol in Particular

In both the short-term and long-term studies it was found that a transient stinging upon instillation was subjectively reported somewhat more frequently by patients with metipranolol than with timolol. A difference in the anaesthetic action of the two substances could not explain this effect. No irritation could be ascertained in tests with the vehicle of the metipranolol eye drops alone, so that this subjective side effect must obviously be produced by the active ingredient itself.

A possibility of avoiding this local side effect was discussed in that for metipranolol the S-isomer of the racemate might be used alone. This idea is based on the assumption that the R-isomer of the racemate which possesses the membrane-stabilizing action, has no pressure-reducing action and that the membrane-stabilizing action might possibly be the cause of these subjective sensations

This principle, i. e. separation of the racemate and use of the S-isomer alone, would, however, only be of practical use if the membrane-stabilizing action does not represent the mechanism of action for the reduction in pressure or does not, even in part, produce a reduction in intraocular pressure.

The decrease in intraocular pressure produced by beta-blocking agents which have no measurable local anaesthetic action, e. g. sotalol and practolol, suggests that the reduction in pressure is due to a specific effect of beta-receptor blockade.

It should be noted that nowadays it is generally assumed that the R- and S-isomers differ from one another by a certain factor with regard to their beta-blocking action, whereby the S-isomer is said to be more effective in its beta-blocking action than the R-isomer by the factor 100. This difference in action, however, depends on the purity of the substance tested. It is now known for some beta-blocking agents which are available in a purer form that the difference in action between the two isomers can be a factor between 200 and 500. It is even probable that the beta-blockade is only present in the left isomeric form and that there is no effective affinity to the beta-receptors at all in the right isomeric form. If there are nevertheless some residues of a beta-blockade to be found in the right isomeric form, this is undoubtedly due to fact that it is chemically impossible to achieve an absolute separation of the isomers. Thus when evaluating data on the difference of action between the two isomers, the purity of the substance tested must be taken into account.

To determine the dependence of subjective complaints on the pH of the eye drops, clinical trials with different solutions of various pH were carried out.

These tests showed that pH higher than 5.5 increasingly produce an extreme instability of the active ingredient. Such pH can, therefore, be used at best for only short periods. In order to test local tolerance, ideal solutions with a short stability and pH of 7.4 were manufactured and instilled. These solutions, however, did not show upon instillation any subjective tolerance other than that of the solution with the pH of 5.5. In this respect it should be remembered that there are also adrenaline preparations which are adjusted to a pH of 2.8 and do not produce subjective complaints. Therefore, it seems that it is not a question of an effect brought about by the pH of the solution, but rather of a property of the active substance itself.

Long-term Medication with Diamox and Beta-Blockers in Combination

From the point of view of the mechanism of action there are obviously two different sites of action. The mechanism on which the action of Diamox is based, i. e. carbonic anhydrase inhibition, is other than that of beta-blocking agents with regard to influencing aqueous production. This seems to be certain. Thus one can assume at least theoretically that a potentiation of action could take place and that both drugs might possibly be a commendable combination. Pertinent reports are to be found in literature. Nevertheless, it must be taken into consideration that it is probably a question of dosage as to whether this combination brings about a further reduction in pressure or not, as both drugs operate predominantly by inhibiting secretion, even if in different ways. On the other hand the aqueous production is controlled in such a manner that a minimum supply always remains guaranteed, i. e. to the extent that nutrition of the lens and the cornea is ensured. The aqueous production is, therefore, not to be limited at will but only to a certain point. If, however, a maximum reduction in aqueous production has already been achieved with one of the two drugs, a further decrease would not be possible by any means.

There are reports in the literature that beta-blocking agents can bring about a further decrease in pressure after medication with Diamox, but again there are others which claim the opposite. As already mentioned, this probably depends on the question of dosage. If all possibilities of limiting aqueous production have not been exhausted, the addition of such a drug may produce a further inhibition in production. On the other hand it is known, however, that also with beta-blocking agents an outflow improving action plays a rôle at least part of the time. This improvement in outflow facility could, of course, bring about a further decrease in pressure. However, this action is possibly not persistent.

Furthermore, there is convincing evidence that a pressure reducing effect by carbonic anhydrase inhibitors is not possible without renal side effects. Therefore, it might well be questioned whether — apart from rare exceptions — it is reasonable nowadays to adjust a patient's intraocular pressure by means of a long-term therapy with Diamox. Studies conducted in large centers in the U. S. A. should be borne in mind: specific questioning of patients undergoing treatment with Diamox showed that the incidence of systemic side effects is between 60 and 70%. Accordingly, there is no long-term reduction in pressure with carbonic anhydrase inhibitors without there being lasting renal effects at the same time and this is not good. For this reason such a therapy should not be considered as a standard long-term therapy.

Comparison of Effects of Metipranolol and Timolol on Ocular Pressure with Particular Reference to Long-term Experience

The phenomenon of hyposensitivity, tolerance or tachyphylaxis — according to time characteristic as it occurs — is non-specific and does not depend on the type of beta-blocking agent. When this phenomenon was first discovered, there was a short interlude during which the existence of the sympton was stubbornly denied, but then an attempt was made to develop a two-phase therapy. This involved alternating a 4-week beta-blocking therapy with a 4-week miotic therapy. It took place at a time when depots similar to Ocusert were being developed and it was found that the process of hyposensitivity was accelerated. This development of tolerance in the eye is non-specific and independent of dose. Accordingly one cannot correct the process of hyposensitivity with more frequent application or with the application of higher concentrations. In serious resistant cases which could not be adjusted with timolol it was seen that the combined administration of timolol and metipranolol at intervals of half an hour did not in any way improve the reduction in pressure.

Side Effects on Functional Capacity and Circulatory Situation of Patients Under Therapy

With regard to the question of systemic side effects of beta-blockers, the initial state of each individual patient must be considered in a differentiated manner. This is a question of the action of the sympatholysis. A sportsman who is dependent on his "sympathetic drive" is less efficient if this is curtailed pharmacologically. In a patient with angina pectoris, in whom this sympathetic drive is rather to be considered as dangerous, the situation is the reverse. In this case performance might even be promoted. This state of affairs must be explained to the patient. Quite generally it can be said that a reduction in efficiency is to be expected sooner in healthy persons than in cardiac patients.

The concentrations of the active ingredient absorbed on topical administration, however, are so small that they are very difficult to detect analytically even with sensitive methods. Therefore, it is also impossible at present to make forecasts or comparisons for the various beta-blocking agents with regard to their potential danger in particularly sensitive patients. Certain absolute and relative contraindications are to be observed for all beta-receptor blocking agents. This includes obstructive airways diseases and also latent heart failure.

As an ophthalmologist one must also bear in mind a general picture of the patient's state when prescribing such drugs.

Depressions as Side Effects Following Local Application of Beta-blocking Agents

In a long-term study no major increase in any type of depression whatsoever was observed in a period of 2 years. Many patients on the other hand showed an improvement in mood because they were happy about the new type of treatment due to the absence of the miotic effect.

The risk of a depression due to therapy with beta-blocking agents can better be assessed in a group of patients that is receiving beta-blocking agents in higher dosage. A clinical trial from the point of view of internal medicine containing a large number of hypertensive cases is available. If one calculates the number of tablets sold and assumes that all these tablets were, in fact, taken, this covers 170,000 patient years. The number of depressions which this group of patients shows is so infinitesimally small that it cannot be given in percentages. The number of official reports on side effects applies to this total number of patients and is four, i. e. not more than four such cases have been reported to the manufacturer.

Allergic Reactions to the Vehicle

The question whether allergic reactions were caused by the vehicle or the active substance in metipranolol eye drops was clarified when the pure vehicle was applied. After the allergic reactions had receded, the pure vehicle was instilled, whereupon the same symptoms occurred as signs of an allergy originating from the vehicle and not the active compound.

But in fact allergic reactions to metipranolol eye drops are extremely few.

Correlation Between the Lipophilia of Drugs and Reduction in Intraocular Pressure

The correlation between the lipophilia of drugs and the reduction in pressure is poor. This is also the reason why pure anaesthetics, for example, do not have any influence at all on intraocular pressure. The problem is that both very lipophilic and very hydrophilic substances have great difficulty in penetrating the cornea and do not at all reach the structures of their site of action, the epithelium of the ciliary body. In order to penetrate the corneal stroma, which is hydrophilic, and the corneal epithelium and corneal endothelium, which are lipophilic, both biophysical properties are necessary. For this reason there is no correlation between one of the properties only and an effect obtained in the interior of the eye.

Dosage and Concentration of Eye Drops

Mishima, who has done much work on the eye in the field of pharmacokinetics, confirms that beta-blocking agents in ophthalmology are hopelessly overdosed. A relative decrease in intraocular pressure of 20—30% can be achieved in long-term therapy, i. e. elevated pressure can be reduced from about 25 to 30 mmHg to 20. This spectrum of elevated intraocular pressure, seen individually, has only a modest damaging value. Therefore, pharmacologists have inhibitions about reducing concentrations of the beta-blockers further and perhaps reaching a lower effect, for it is not very relevant to decrease pressure from 23 to 20. As the risk of damage increases exponentially with the increase in pressure, a patient with an intraocular pressure of 28 might well run 20 times more risk of damage than that of a patient with 24 mmHg.

If one approaches the minimum clinically effective dose, the long-term effect proves to be too slight. Therefore, we achieve efficacy for a long-term period by a supramaximal active concentration; to be sure, we have no better effects due to the higher dosage but we do bring about the long-term efficacy and thus make it possible for instillation to be only once or twice daily. Theoretically, one could achieve this with significantly lower concentrations applied several times.

However, this could require the patients' collaboration. There are studies which, in fact, show that timolol applied twice daily does not reduce pressure to a significantly greater extent than when applied once daily. There is a slight difference but this is, as already said, not significant. An attempt seems commendable to test lower concentrations of the active ingredient as can be seen in another marketed form of beta-blocking agent which has now been introduced to the German market with a more moderate dosage. Another question is whether it might not be more expedient to decrease the amount of the dose by making the size of the drops smaller. This seems to be an interesting aspect, as the total volume of the liquid in the region of the palpebral fissure is about 8—10 microliters and, basically, with a volume per drop of 50 microliters too much substance and liquid is applied to the eye. The problem to be resolved is how to make it clinically possible to find an applicator that instils very small volumes of drops. This justifies the hope of having a decrease in side effects due to a reduction in the quantity applied. Theoretically, one can obtain about 30 drops from 1 ml. Not the viscosity of the substance but the surface tension is decisive for the volume of a drop. This may possibly be influenced by the inclusion of preservatives.

On no account, however, can the volume of the drop be varied by changing the viscosity or possibly by changing the aperture of the dropper bottle.

Sicca Syndrome and Topical Beta-blocking Therapy

The triggering off of a sicca syndrome due to topical beta-blocking therapy does not seem very probable. Rather an additive effect in the case of already existing topical diseases is to be expected.

An increase in an already existing sicca syndrome or intensification of paretic corneal disorders also seems conceivable, whereby we have impediments in the axoplasmatic flow.

Recommendations for Future Research in Conservative Glaucoma Therapy, Particularly in Therapy with Beta-blockers

There are concrete ideas which, in part, are already under study. The main point of interest is beta-blocking agents that have a significantly lower membrane-stabilizing or anaesthetic action than all others hitherto. Particularly attention is also be paid to the question of concentration which can evidently be considerably reduced in some products; the investigation of this is, however, still at a very early stage. The question of the isomer, in particular which advantages the S-isomer might have, has already been discussed in detail. If the intraocular pressure lowering effect is, however, not bound at all to the beta-blocker, then the consequences would be considerable, namely this would offer the R-isomer the advantage that systemic side effects in the sense of asthmatic provocation would no longer occur.

Another idea worth considering in this connection might be vaso-dilating beta-blocker agents. Here also there is a number of new substances, e. g. prizidilol, carvedilol (BM 14 190), BM 12 434. These are products which probably do not cause deficiency in blood supply, as is normally expected of beta-blocking agents. The question, however, is whether these substances still have an intraocular pressure reducing effect at all. It may possibly be that they no longer possess the property of inhibiting aqueous production.

Another possibility of improving beta-blocking agents might be the joining of these substances to acids as e. g. with propranolol hemisuccinate. This could possibly achieve a better penetration, a reduction in dosage and an increase in action — even if attempts in the manufacturing of other substances — as we know to be the case for dipivalylepinephrine — have so far produced negative results in trials.

Corneal Sensitivity
Measurement and Clinical Importance

By J. Draeger

with the collaboration of **M. Ackermann, H. Buhr-Unger, K. Hanke, K. Karjalainen, C. C. Kok-van-Alphen, H. Langenbucher, M. Lüders, R. Martin, B. Riss, E. Rumberger, W. Schloot, H. J. Völker-Dieben, R. Winter**

Translated from the German by **F. C. Blodi**

1984. Approx. 90 figures. Approx. 160 pages.
Cloth DM 69,-, öS 484,-. ISBN 3-211-81794-8

Prices are subject to change without notice

The sensitivity of the cornea elicits one of the most delicate defense reflexes of the human body. That is why early and diagnostically significant recognition of pathological changes is possible here. Now modern microprocessor technology has succeeded in developing a highly sensitive apparatus for quick and quantitatively reproducible measurement of corneal sensitivity.

This opens a wide field for experimental and clinical investigation. Some of the many topics concerned are: differential diagnosis and control of the course of herpetic diseases of the cornea; reinnervation following surgical intervention in the anterior section of the eye; effects of various beta-blockers on the cornea; basic questions of tolerance and adaptive quality of contact lenses; and the dimensions of damage caused by glaucoma, elucidated by the direct correlation between disturbed sensitivity and stage of the glaucoma. Thus a new era of ophthalmologic examination and diagnostics has begun, whose consequences are not fully assessable yet. This book covers not only the physiological basis, operating method and potential of the apparatus; it also gives—for the calibration of actually measured values—an outline of threshold values of corneal sensitivity.

Springer-Verlag Wien New York

Corneal Sensitivity

Measurement and Clinical Importance

Springer-Verlag Wien New York